"*The Happiest Baby on the Block* presents the top science about the development of babies. It will guide new parents for many years to come."

—JULIUS RICHMOND, M.D., former U.S. Surgeon General

"This is the best way I know to help crying babies."

—STEVEN SHELOV, M.D., editor in chief, American Academy of Pediatrics' *Caring for Your New Baby and Young Child: Birth to Age Five*

"*The Happiest Baby on the Block* is fun and convincing. I highly recommend it."

—ELISABETH BING, co-founder, Lamaze International

"Dr. Karp has written the best book that I've read on this challenging topic."

—MORRIS GREEN, M.D., director, Behavioral Pediatrics, Indiana University School of Medicine

"What a marvelous book! Parents for years to come will be grateful to Dr. Karp for this lucid and entertaining explanation of why babies cry and how to help them."

—MARTIN STEIN, M.D., professor of pediatrics, University of California, San Diego Medical School; co-author of *Encounters with Children: Pediatric Behavior and Development*

Celebrities Praise

The Happiest Baby

"A must read! Dr. Karp offers insights into parenting by combining ancient and modern wisdom. Our baby boy responded to the 5 S's immediately!"

—KEELY AND PIERCE BROSNAN, TV journalist/
environmentalist and actor

"There is nothing quite like watching Dr. Harvey work wonders on a screaming baby. He's not a pediatrician; he's a magician. Every time I bring my kids in to see him, I walk out wishing he was their father."

—LARRY DAVID, star of *Curb Your Enthusiasm*
and co-creator of *Seinfeld*

"What every mother needs are simple tools that really work . . . and Harvey's do."

—MICHELLE PFEIFFER, actress/producer

"Now babies and toddlers—and their parents—can sleep better and longer thanks to Dr. Karp's practical advice and wisdom."

—ARIANNA HUFFINGTON, editor in chief, *The Huffington Post*

"When I was bone tired from my little boy's sleep struggles, I turned to the top sleep guru for modern moms, Dr. Harvey Karp."

—TINA SHARKEY, chairman and global president,
BabyCenter.com

"Harvey Karp would make my Big Mama proud! He is leading us back to age-old basics, back to motherwit."

—ALFRE WOODARD, actress

"Harvey Karp's enlightened and creative approach has been a benefit not only to our children, but to my wife and me as parents."

—LINDSEY BUCKINGHAM, photographer and singer/
songwriter, Fleetwood Mac

"Dr. Karp was exactly the doctor to see us through new parenthood. He has the magic touch—not just with babies, but with new parents, too."

—ROBIN SWICORD, screenwriter, *Matilda* and
Memoirs of a Geisha

"Dr. Karp is simply the best. Anytime our kids have a problem, he guides us with warmth, wisdom, and humor."

—JANET AND JERRY ZUCKER, director, *Airplane,*
The Naked Gun, and *Rat Race*

Parents Praise

The Happiest Baby

"I'll give you $100 if you teach me what you just did to calm my baby."

—DENISE, MICHAEL, JACQUELINE, AND OLIVIA

"Curtis's crying was loud and piercing. The only thing I have found to calm him were those 'tricks' you teach in your office."

—CAROL, DON, CURTIS, AND CARTER

"Our daughter cried terribly. Exhausted, I went to see Dr. Karp. After using his technique, we became believers. Incredibly, it always works for us."

—ALISE, WILL, AND CAMERON

"We owe you our second born for teaching us 'The Karp.' It's a miracle cure for colic!"

—ANA, JEFF, AND ALEXANDER

"We call it the 'Harvey Shuffle.' The first time I saw it I was astounded. In seconds, Ben stopped crying and my jaw was on the floor!"

—CHRISTINA, JONAH, AND BEN

"My wife and I bought no less than ten baby books. But the things you showed us were not in the books."

—MARTIN, ANN, AND MADISON

"Swaddling Theo made a huge difference. Now he is sleeping five to six hours straight at night. It even stopped his spitting up at night. We owe you."

—LISA, EVAN, AND THEO

"Dr. Karp's method was a lifesaver. With a simple 1, 2, 3—swaddle, shhhh, swing—our baby fell asleep and we received a round of applause."

—LAUREL, ATILLIO, RAFFAELLA, AND ROCCO

"Colic hit us like a freight train. I called Dr. Karp and within two weeks, Emma was sleeping eight to ten hours a night. Dr. Karp changed our lives!"

—JODY, SAM, AND EMMA

BY HARVEY KARP, M.D.

The Happiest Baby on the Block (book and DVD)
The Happiest Toddler on the Block (book and DVD)
The Happiest Baby Guide to Great Sleep

The Happiest Baby on the Block

SECOND EDITION

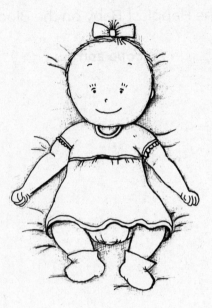

BANTAM BOOKS | NEW YORK

The Happiest Baby on the Block

The New Way to Calm Crying and

Help Your Newborn Baby

Sleep Longer

SECOND EDITION

Harvey Karp, M.D.

2015 Bantam Books Revised Trade Paperback Edition

Copyright © 2002, 2015 by The Happiest Baby, Inc.
Illustrations by Jennifer Kalis, copyright © 2002 The Happiest Baby, Inc.

Published in the United States by Bantam Books, an imprint of Random House,
a division of Penguin Random House LLC, New York.

BANTAM BOOKS and the HOUSE colophon are registered trademarks of
Penguin Random House LLC.

"The Happiest Baby on the Block" and "The 5 S's" are registered trademarks of
The Happiest Baby, Inc.

Originally published in hardcover and in different form in the United States
by Bantam Books, an imprint of Random House,
a division of Penguin Random House LLC, in 2002.

LIBRARY OF CONGRESS CATALOGING-IN-PUBLICATION DATA
Karp, Harvey.
The happiest baby on the block : the new way to calm crying and help your newborn baby
sleep longer / Harvey Karp, M.D.—Second edition.
pages   cm
Includes bibliographical references and index.
ISBN 978-0-553-39323-1 (paperback)
ISBN 978-0-8041-7997-3 (ebook)
1. Crying in infants.   2. Infants—Care.   3. Parent and child.
4. Infants—Sleep.   5. Child rearing.   I. Title.
RJ253.K37 2015
649'.122—dc23   2015012546

Printed in the United States of America on acid-free paper

randomhousebooks.com

12 14 16 18 19 17 15 13

Book design by Mary A. Wirth

*To the generous hearts
of new parents everywhere.
And to our sweet babies
who come into the world
with such trust.*

CONTENTS

~~~~~~~~~~~~~~~

ACKNOWLEDGMENTS

"One's mind, once stretched by a new idea, never regains its original dimensions."

—OLIVER WENDELL HOLMES SR.

I am a pediatrician—and I love it. I am privileged to practice a field of medicine where I get to be part biologist, part psychologist, part anthropologist, part animal impersonator, and even part grandmother.

In this book, I also wear all those hats. My greatest goal is to use all those skills to share with parents, grandparents—and everyone who cares about babies—how to translate their messages of love into the language all babies understand.

This book took years to prepare and would never have been completed without the encouragement of a small group of family, friends, and colleagues, to whom I owe my profound gratitude:

- To my beloved mother, Sophie, who taught me to marvel at the beauty and order in the world, and to my father, Joe, whose patience is my model and whose selfless generosity sheltered me and gave me the gift of education.

- To my extraordinary wife, Nina, my soul mate, who opened my heart and eyes and is my greatest friend, teacher, and compass. To my mother-in-law, Desa, who was a unique and courageous woman. And to my daughter, Lexi, who graciously tolerated my long hours of work.

- To my great (and growing) team: Marija Sipka, Kelly Nielson, Roy Kosuge, Steve Hecker, Jovo Majstorovic, Neal Tabachnick, Louise Teeter, Yves Behar and the Fuseproject team, Deb Roy, Rupal Patel, Loree Stringer, Matt Berlin and Jesse Gray, Bill Washabaugh, Ted Larson, Sharon Fox, Zack Exley, and Tony Donofrio.

- To my teacher Arthur H. Parmelee, Jr., whose brilliant talent for making the complex seem simple helped me learn how to observe and understand children.

- To the curious minds of Julius Richmond, T. Berry Brazelton, Tiffany Field, Brad Thach, Fern Hauck, Rachel Moon, Rosemary Horne, Peter Blair, Ronald Barr, Ian St. James-Roberts, and many other honest explorers of science whose road signs guided me on this wonderful path into the inner world of babies.

- To the doctors and friends who so generously read, reviewed, and tested out my work: Julius Richmond, Steven Shelov, Jim Hmurovic, Arianna Huffington, William Coleman, Morris Green, Lewis Leavitt, Stanley Inkelis, Neal and Fran Kaufman, Roni Cohen Leiderman, James McKenna, Barton Schmitt, Elisabeth Bing, Julee Waldrop, Teresa Olsen, Ann Kellams, Marty Stein, Anne Grauer, Tina Sharkey, Keely and Pierce Brosnan, Madonna, Michelle Pfeiffer, Larry David, Alfre Woodard, Hunter Tylo, Robin Swicord and Nick Kazan, Jerry and Janet Zucker, Kristen and Lindsay Buckingham, Toby Berlin and Michael Grecco, Laurie David, Eric Weissler, Richard Grant, Sylvie Rabineau, Katy Arnoldi, Laurel and Tom Barrack, Jonathan Feldman, Dick and Lïse Stolley, Carrie Cook, and my partners and staff at Tenth Street, whose support helped make this work possible.

- To the many doctors and researchers who have invested their time and efforts in studying the 5 S's work: Manjusha Abraham, Argelinda Baroni, Erika Bocknek, Ruben Fukkink, Margreet Harskamp van Ginkel, Christopher Greeley, John Harrington, Sarah Hoehn, Deepak Kamat, Carole Lesham, Maria Muzik, Nicole Miller, Joanna Parga, Ian Paul, Heather Risser, Roos Rodenburg, Robert Sege, Martine Stikkelorum, Benjamin Van Voorhees, and Lonnie Zeltzer.
- To the hundreds of parenting leaders around the world who have been invaluable allies in bringing these messages to parents: Laura Jana, Martha Kautz, Julie Shaffer, Michelle Saysana, Jennifer Shu, Barton Schmitt, Anita Berry, Sherry Iverson, Sherry Bonnes, Matthew Melmed, Chris Lester, Jetta Bernier, Don Middleton, and many, many more.
- To the thousands of certified *Happiest Baby* educators giving skills and confidence to new parents in universities, hospitals, public health programs, military bases, prisons, teen parenting programs, and so forth across the United States and around the world.
- To the great team at Penguin Random House, from the sharp intellect of my editor, Marnie Cochran, to the witty imagination of my illustrator, Jennifer Kalis, and to the savvy advice of my agent, Suzanne Gluck.
- And, most of all, my profound thanks go to all the parents who have taken these ideas to heart and shared the 5 S's with their friends and family. It gives me the greatest joy when a mom or dad tells me that they learned about *The Happiest Baby* from a buddy on the assembly line, a pastor at church, parents they met on the playground . . . and even from total strangers.

Thank you all!

INTRODUCTION

~~~~~~~~~~~~~

Ancient Secrets About Crying Babies

When I started medical school, I was taught that when babies scream it's a sign of gas pain. And there were two approaches to soothe them: natural (holding, rocking, pacifiers) and medical (sedatives, antispasm syrups, or gas drops). Unfortunately, the natural ways failed 20 percent of the time, and the medical approach was often useless or led to serious problems (sedating was inappropriate; antispasm drugs caused coma and death; gas drops were no more effective than plain water).

By 1978, I was a fully trained pediatrician, yet I was totally helpless caring for colicky babies. And soon, my helplessness turned into shock and alarm. While working on the child abuse team at UCLA, I saw babies who were severely injured—even killed—for the simple offense of crying. But please don't think the mothers and fathers who hurt their babies were mean, terrible people. For the most part, they were just exhausted and stressed-out young parents who cracked under the strain of their baby's unstoppable shrieks.

Puzzled why advanced science hadn't yet solved the common—

yet disturbing—problem of colic, I began to read everything I could, searching for clues to solve this mysterious condition. I soon uncovered two facts that turned my alarm into hope.

First, I learned about the profound leap in brain development that occurs between birth and four months. In a brilliant report by one of America's top pediatricians, Arthur H. Parmelee, Jr., he observed that many parents naively expect their baby to be born smiling and interactive. And they're often shocked when they're handed a "fetus-like" newborn whose shrieks could shatter glass.

My second realization came when I began to study how parents in other societies raised their children. Delving through the musty books and journals at the UCLA library, I was shocked to learn that colicky screaming was virtually absent in at least one culture!

It became apparent to me that our culture—advanced in so many ways—was backward when it came to baby soothing. I discovered that our practices were based on centuries of myths and misconceptions. Suddenly, it was clear that this confounding puzzle—"Why do some babies cry so much?"—had a simple but odd solution: *Babies cry because they're born three months too soon!*

Of course, I've never talked a mom into carrying her baby for three extra months. But, compared to baby horses or cows, it's obvious our babies are not ready *to come out of the oven after just nine months.* I'm confident that you'll notice

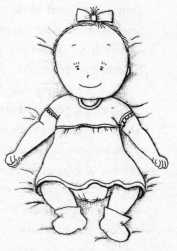

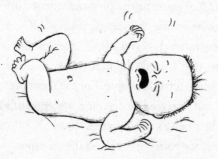

how your newborn loves womb-like holding, rocking, and skin-to-skin touch.

But *why* is imitating the womb so calming? And why does it work for some babies but fail for others? These questions led to a new idea: Rhythmic, womb-like sound, motion, and touch must trigger an automatic *reflex* . . . but this calming reflex only works if done exactly right.

This idea of a calming reflex explained the well-known observation that the world's best baby calmers succeed by giving babies rhythmic sensations. And it explained why bouncy car rides and rumbling hair dryer sounds often quiet screams in a snap. It even solved other ancient riddles, like why adults find rocking in hammocks so soothing, why we're calmed by the sound of the ocean and rain, why we fall asleep in cars and planes, and why even an upset ninety-two-year-old feels more at peace when she is rocked, held, and shushed. All are tied to our powerfully soothing experiences in utero.

Studying calming tricks used around the world, I found most fit into five simple steps: swaddling, the side/stomach position, shushing, swinging, and sucking. I call these the 5 S's.

For thousands of years, the most skilled parents have used the 5 S's to soothe their babies, and soon you'll be an expert at them, too!

Note: If your baby is very fussy, feel free to skip ahead and dive right into the discussion about exactly how to do the 5 S's, starting with chapter 8. Otherwise, I invite you to join me on a little journey—from ancient times to the twenty-first century—to see how newborns experience the world and to learn how to calm your baby's crying—and boost sleep—usually in just days.

PART ONE

Why Babies Cry, and Why Some Cry So Much

1

~~~~~

Babies: A New Insight

MAIN POINTS

- All babies cry, but most new parents have little experience soothing them.
- The missing fourth trimester: Babies cry because they're born three months too soon!
- The calming reflex: Nature's brilliant "off switch" for your baby's crying.
- The 5 S's: Five simple steps to imitate the womb and turn on the calming reflex.
- The Cuddle Cure: Comforting your baby with his/her preferred mix of S's.

Suzanne was freaking out. Her two-month-old was a nonstop screamer. Sean could cry for hours—even through the night—and his mother was desperately exhausted. One afternoon her sister, Angie, visited to help. As soon as Angie picked Sean up,

Suzanne bolted to the bathroom for a hot shower. Twenty-five minutes later, she awoke, curled in a ball on the shower's blue tile floor, being sprayed with ice-cold water.

While this was happening in California, on the plains of Botswana, Nisa nursed her baby, Chuko. Chuko was delicate and small, but she rarely cried for more than a few seconds.

Nisa carried Chuko everywhere in a leather sling. She never worried when Chuko cried, because—having cared for so many little cousins—she knew exactly how to calm her.

Why did Suzanne fail at soothing Sean's screams? And what secrets did Nisa know that settled Chuko so quickly?

YOUR BABY IS BORN

When perfectly dry, his flesh sweet and pure, he is the most kissable object in nature.

Marion Harland, *Common Sense in the Nursery*, 1886

If you're pregnant or have a new baby, *congratulations!* Having a baby is a wonderful—and wonder-filled—experience that makes us laugh, cry, and stare in amazement . . . all at the same time. It's a miraculous and profound life event that can make gamblers give up gambling, drug addicts stop getting high, and hard-core bikers buy minivans!

After giving birth, your top jobs for the next few months will be feeding your baby well and calming her cries. After thirty years as a pediatrician, I can tell you that parents who succeed at these tasks feel proud and confident. However, parents who struggle with them feel distraught and incompetent.

Fortunately, baby feeding is usually pretty easy. Most newborns happily gulp down the milk as if you were a five-star restaurant. And if you run into difficulties, there are many places to turn for help. Soothing crying, on the other hand, can be unexpectedly hard.

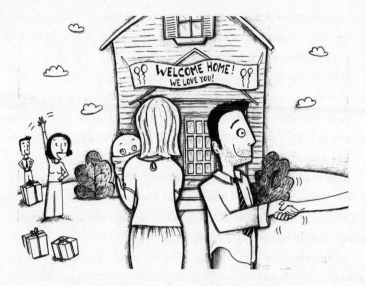

No couple expects their sweet newborn to be "difficult." (Your friends may share horror stories about screaming babies, but most of us think, *That won't be my child!*) So we're usually shocked when our little one's wails go on and on no matter what we do.

Now, I'm not saying crying is bad. In fact, it's brilliant! Leave it to nature to equip helpless babies with a way to make even the most exhausted mom vault out of a warm bed—on a cold night—and hustle over to meet her little one's needs.

Once your *fusser* has your attention, you'll want to zip through a short checklist:

- If she's hungry . . . feed her.
- If she's wet . . . change her diaper.
- If she's cold . . . bundle her up.
- If she's hot . . . unwrap her.
- If she's lonely . . . pick her up.

The trouble comes when none of these steps works.

Fifty percent of babies have bouts of inconsolable fussiness lasting two hours a day—or more. And 10–15 percent—about half a million new babies born each year—suffer three-*plus* hours of red-faced, eye-clenched screaming a day.

This is why new parents are such heroes!

A baby's scream is heart-wrenching. And hours of inconsolable crying can trigger a panic of self-doubt: "Is my baby in pain?" "Does she hate me?" "Am I spoiling her?" "Does she feel abandoned?" "Am I a terrible mother?"

Distraught parents are often counseled that there's no cure for fussy, sleepless babies. They are told they must wait a few months for their baby to "grow out of it." Yet, it feels like *torture* to sit by while your baby cries and cries.

Confronted by this barrage, even the most loving parents may get pushed into waves of anxiety, depression, or the tragedies of suicide or child abuse.

Note: I've been told that Navy SEALS are trained to endure severe sleep deprivation *and hours of infant crying blasted over loud speakers.* In other words, the military prepares warriors to handle torture by exposing them to . . . a typical day in the life of a new mom or dad!

HELP WANTED: WHERE DO PARENTS TURN WHEN THEIR BABY CRIES A LOT?

Today's moms and dads are among the most educated parents who ever lived. But when it comes to babies, they have less experience than any generation in history! Shockingly, we're required to have more preparation and training to get a driver's license than to have a baby.

Of course, regardless of your training, you should still expect to be the target of an onslaught of advice. Family, friends—even total strangers—shower us with their counsel. "It's boredom." "It's the heat." "Put a hat on him." "It's gas." I think America's favorite pastime isn't baseball. . . . It's giving new moms unsolicited advice.

And advice is something parents of fussy babies definitely need. One in six couples takes their baby to the doctor because of persistent crying. Yet, while thousands of clinics have been created to solve feeding problems, very few are set up to help with screaming babies. In fact, most doctors have little to offer families of colicky babies, other than sympathy. "I know it's hard, but be patient; it won't last forever." Or, even worse, "Just put your baby in a dark room and let her cry. She just needs to blow off steam." (*Hey, babies aren't pressure cookers.*)

Top baby experts usually confess that they have few tools to help really fussy babies:

> *Very often, you may not even be able to quiet the screaming.*
>
> Heidi Eisenberg Murkoff, Arlene Eisenberg, Sandee E. Hathaway, and Sharon Mazel, *What to Expect the First Year*

> *The whole episode goes on at least an hour and perhaps for three or four hours.*
>
> Penelope Leach, *Your Baby and Child*

> *Crying up to* five hours *a day is not unusual. When you begin to become very frustrated with a baby's crying, it is time to set the infant in a safe place and walk away.*
>
> Period of PURPLE Crying program

Well, it turns out that these ideas are all obsolete. Screaming does not have to go on for hours. And what's even more concerning, when left unchecked, nonstop crying can trigger serious problems, like postpartum depression, crib death (from unsafe sleeping practices), and failed breast-feeding.

Of course, if your patience is frayed and you fear you might hurt your child, *you must put her down . . . take a break . . . and call a friend for help.* But if a mom in the wilds of Africa can calm her baby in under a minute, you can bet that there's probably a way to help unhappy babies in our culture, too.

THE FOUR PRINCIPLES OF BABY SOOTHING

Botswanan moms carry their infants in leather sacks twenty-four hours a day (cuddling and bouncing as they walk). They also calm their infants by nursing them fifty to a hundred times a day . . . including all through the night! You may not be ready to adopt the Botswana lifestyle, but the key lesson of their success is that *colic is not inevitable.* Persistent crying is an unintended side effect of our culture. However, the good news is that, with the right techniques, we, too, can calm most screaming bouts in under one minute.

By teasing out shreds of wisdom from past cultures and weaving them with modern research, I've found that the key to calming crying and boosting sleep can be explained through four simple ideas:

- The missing fourth trimester
- The calming reflex
- The 5 S's
- The Cuddle Cure

The Missing Fourth Trimester: Babies Cry Because They're Born Too Soon!

Baby cows, camels, and horses can walk—even run—on their first days of life. In fact, they must be able to run. Those who can't are quickly eaten by predators.

By comparison, our newborns are super immature. They can't run . . . walk . . . or even burp without our help. One British mum said her baby seemed so unready for the world she nicknamed her "the Little Creature." And she was not alone in viewing babies that way; the Spanish sometimes call newborns *criaturas,* meaning "creatures."

I find it most helpful to think of new babies as being mushy, smushy *fetuses. Imagine this:* Had your labor been three months longer, your baby would have been born smiling, cooing, and flirting with you. (Who wouldn't want *that* on the first day of life!) Of course, no woman can actually do that. At nine months, getting the baby's head out is already a very tight squeeze, and by twelve months it would be impossible.

So the answer to the question "Why are our babies so immature at birth?" is quite simple: Unlike a baby horse—whose survival depends on having a big, strong body—a human child's survival depends on having a big, smart brain. In fact, the brain is so huge that babies have to be "evicted" from the womb well before they're fully "baked." Otherwise, the head might get stuck coming through the tight birth canal, killing both mother and baby.

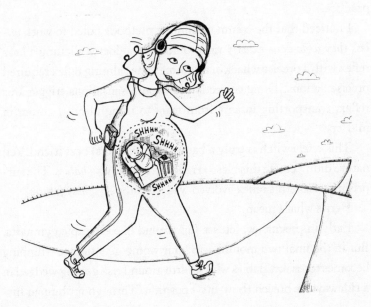

We know that, for thousands of years, parents have intuitively understood this. That's why, from swaddling to swinging to shushing, almost every traditional baby-calming technique returns babies to that cuddly, rhythmic prenatal world.

This fourth trimester is a pleasant comfort for easy babies, but it is *absolutely essential* for fussy ones. Yet, surprisingly, rocking and shushing don't work by making babies feel "back home." Imitating the womb actually works by triggering a calming reflex, a profound and ancient neurological response deep in the baby's brain.

The Calming Reflex: Nature's Brilliant "Off Switch" for Your Baby's Crying

For thousands of years, experienced moms and grandmas have intuitively rocked and shushed babies to soothe them. But the recognition that these sensations flipped on a calming reflex was completely overlooked until the mid-1990s, when I stumbled upon the idea while working with hundreds of crying babies in my practice.

I noticed that the common calming methods failed to work *unless they were done exactly right*. Similar to a doctor eliciting a *knee* reflex with a precise whack of a hammer, the calming reflex required precise actions. Done correctly, the womb sensations trigger this reflex, transporting infants from tears to tranquility . . . often in mid-cry.

This *reset* switch is truly a baby's (and parent's) best friend. Yet, nature didn't create this blessed reflex to calm *crying babies*. The surprising reason this reflex evolved was to soothe . . . *fussy fetuses!*

Here's what I mean:

Early in pregnancy, fetuses flip around like Olympic gymnasts. But in the final two months—as your womb gets tighter—flipping becomes too risky. Babies who squirm around risk getting wedged in a sideways or breech (butt-first) position. Throughout human history breech babies often got stuck coming down the birth canal. That terrible event usually killed both the baby and the mother. (That's exactly how my wife's grandmother died.)

But over millennia, fetuses developed a new talent. During the last months of pregnancy, they became hypnotized by the rhythmic sounds and motions of the womb. This kept these Zen little babies resting—in the safer head-down position—just waiting to be born. It's possible that the survival of our species was possible only because of this ancient calming reflex.

The 5 S's: Five Steps to Turn On Your Baby's Calming Reflex

We don't have kangaroo pouches for our immature newborns to hop back into. But we *do* have arms, swaddling blankets, and slings to surround our little *criaturas* with sensations that magically entranced them in the womb during the final months of pregnancy.

To create a fourth trimester of perfect "wombness," we need to know the details: What *exactly* is it like inside there?

Well, inside you, your baby is tightly packed into the fetal position; constantly embraced/massaged by the warm, velvet wall of the womb; and rocked and jiggled for much of the day. But what is surprising is that they are also surrounded by a constant, rumbly shush . . . that is louder than a vacuum cleaner.

Knowing this clarifies why babies are soothed by experiences, such as hair dryers, car rides, and white noise downloads. And it sheds light on why most traditional baby-calming techniques imitate five universal womb sensations:

1. **SWADDLING:** Snug wrapping
2. **SIDE/STOMACH:** Lying on the side or stomach (only when you are there with your baby; never for sleep)
3. **SHUSHING:** Strong white noise

4. SWINGING: Tiny rhythmic, jiggly motions (just one inch, back and forth)

5. SUCKING: Sucking on your nipple, a clean finger, or a pacifier

These steps may not sound very innovative, but what *is* revolutionary is that—when done *exactly* right—these steps (called the 5 S's) usually settle baby screams in seconds. (And, when done incorrectly, they do nothing . . . or even cause *more* crying!) Detailed descriptions of how to perfectly perform each S are found in chapters 8 through 12.

The Cuddle Cure: Finding Your Baby's Perfect Mix of S's

Knowing each S may not be enough to calm your baby. Think of it like baking a cake. To be successful you need to know much more than the ingredients in the recipe. You must know how much of each to use, how to grease the pan, or how hot the oven should be. Knowing only the ingredients, but not how to prepare them, you're more likely to end up with a bunch of goop than a perfect cake.

Similarly, fussy babies only calm when the S's are done correctly and when three, four, or five of the S's are all done at the same time. (A mom in my practice dubbed combining several S's together the Cuddle Cure.)

The starting point of calming is usually snug wrapping, or swaddling. Indeed, if baby calming were a layer cake, swaddling would be the first layer. It keeps babies from flailing and making themselves even more upset.

Note: Swaddling by itself often fails to calm fussing, but it prepares your baby to focus on the next "layers" you add . . . which *will* turn on the calming reflex.

Next comes the side/stomach position. The back is the only safe position when you place your baby down, but it usually worsens crying . . . making them feel that they're falling. The side or stomach

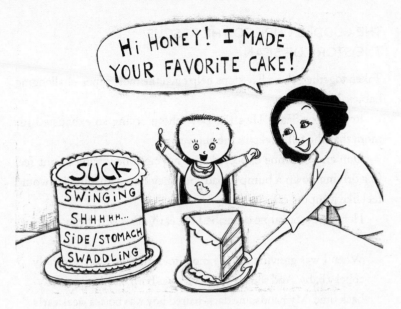

creates a sense of safety, and for many babies it's super-effective at turning on the calming reflex. The next two layers are shushing and swinging. Both are potent triggers of the calming reflex. They relax your baby so she can escape the cycle of crying and notice all your wonderful cuddling and feeding. Last, but not least, sucking is the icing on the cake. It keeps the calming reflex turned on and gives infants a profound sense of peace.

Note: Sucking—all by itself—can sometimes stop a baby's upset in mid-wail. But, if that fails, just swaddle and start layering on the other steps.

Each baby is an individual, with his or her own preferences. But, with a bit of practice, you'll soon discover the mix and intensity of the 5 S's that your baby likes the best.

THE CUDDLE CURE TO THE RESCUE:
THE STORY OF SEAN

Taken together, these five steps help even the most super-challenging babies, like Sean.

Remember Sean? He's the boy whose crying so exhausted his mom that she fell asleep in the shower.

Don and Suzanne expected that having a new baby might feel like driving down a bumpy road, but they never imagined it would feel like jumping off a cliff!

Here's how Suzanne described the early days with Sean:

When I was growing up, my mom told me that I was a terribly colicky baby. And shortly after Sean was born, I knew it was pay-back time. My handsome dark-haired boy was born a week early but, like a racehorse, he was "out of the gate" at a gallop!

From the second week of life, Sean had uncontrollable screaming for hours every day. I felt like a failure as I watched him writhe in pain. Nothing helped and I usually ended up crying right along with him.

Equally devastating was my secret fear that Sean's cries were the result of some injury he suffered at birth. His delivery was difficult. After two hours of hard pushing, the obstetrician yanked him out with vacuum suction. My first memory of Sean is seeing his poor head looking like a black and blue banana.

During the early weeks, our pediatrician said the wailing was just his need to "blow off steam." He warned that responding too fast would spoil him and teach him to cry even more. That sounded logical, but leaving Sean made him shriek even more—plus it was agonizing for us.

Don and I sought every bit of advice we could find. Day after day, we tried new remedies: swaddling—a failure; pacifier—useless; a change in my diet—futile; a swing—like waving to a jet thirty thousand feet overhead. We even tried a device that imitated a car's noise and vibration. That was a bust, too.

Exhausted and demoralized, we returned to our doctor. He sympathetically repeated that we had no option other than to endure Sean's shrieking until he outgrew this phase. That afternoon, Don and I agreed that it would be unbearable to wait.

At our wits' end, we took our six-week-old to a new pediatrician. He asked us many questions, and once he was convinced that Sean's crying wasn't a serious medical condition, he taught us the 5 S's.

The doctor said most babies cry because they're just not ready to be born. They need the protected world of the uterus for another three months!

To be honest, I thought, this is way too simple to be true. After all, I had tried wrapping, rocking, and white noise and ended up as squashed as a bug under a flyswatter. But after watching his demonstration I realized I was doing them wrong.

Don and I decided to try everything again. As incredible as it sounds, that afternoon was the last time Sean cried uncontrollably.

We were ecstatic that we had finally found the comfort Sean had needed for so many weeks. From that day on, whenever he began going berserk, we would do all the steps, and his little body would almost always relax and melt into our arms . . . in under a minute.

Note: It's hard to learn anything new when someone is "yelling at you." That's why it's best to practice the 5 S's when your baby is calm. Parents who follow the techniques exactly as described in the book usually master them within five to ten tries.

Some parents hesitate using the 5 S's. They've heard swaddling is bad for nursing; or shushing is bad for hearing; or responding to every cry creates bad habits. Thankfully, all those worries are unfounded. Hours of motion, sound, and snug cuddling give infants the entrancing help they need to handle the chaos of colors, faces, sounds, and smells they now experience throughout their waking hours.

By four months your baby will be much better at calming herself with cooing, moving, and finger sucking. More on that later.

PARENTING CRYING BABIES ... IN THE TWENTY-FIRST CENTURY

I hope you're excited to learn these steps. It's my hope that this knowledge will be shared—from parent to parent—until, one day, colic will only be found in dictionaries.

By the time you finish the book, I hope you will feel totally confident with the 5 S's. I believe it will help you stop many hours of screaming and add many hours of sleep.

The rest of part one of the book will detail:

• Why do babies cry?
• What is colic and how can you tell if your baby has it?
• Why do gas pains, immaturity, a baby's temperament, and mom's anxiety *rarely* cause colic?
• What is the true cause of colic?

And part two will explain:

• How to do each of the 5 S's
• How to mix the different S's to get the best, fastest results
• Other baby-soothing ideas
• Tricks and tips to boost your infant's sleep
• The few medical problems that can cause colic

You've been blessed with one of life's most amazing experiences—the birth of a baby. So strap yourself in and enjoy the ride. And when your baby cries consider it an opportunity to perfect your new skills as you learn how to turn your fussy infant into *the happiest baby on your block*!

Note: If you have a very fussy baby and need to learn the 5 *S's right now,* feel free to jump ahead to chapter 8.

2

~~~~~~

Crying: Our Infants' Ancient
Survival Tool

MAIN POINTS

- The *crying reflex:* Your baby's brilliant attention-getting tool.
- Crying works by making us want to respond immediately.
- Whimper! Cry! Shriek!: Your baby's three-word vocabulary.

> *A baby's cry . . . cries to be turned off.*
>
> Peter Ostwald, *Soundmaking: The Acoustic*
> *Communication of Emotion*

At birth, your newborn's powerful wails are a welcome sign that he is healthy.

Be grateful for your baby's ability to cry! Getting a parent's attention is so important that babies are equipped with the ability to cry from the first moment of life. During the first months, crying helps your newborn get everything he needs without the foggiest idea of how to ask for it. In fact, he would be in terrible danger if he couldn't call out to you.

THE *CRYING REFLEX:* THE BRILLIANT WAY TINY BABIES GET THEIR MOM'S ATTENTION

All baby animals need to get their mom's attention, but few of them would ever scream for it. Loud sounds could be fatal for a puppy or a young rabbit, because it would reveal their location to a hungry predator. That's why needy kittens meekly meow, monkeys softly beep, and baby gorillas barely whimper.

Human newborns, on the other hand, abandoned such quiet caution long ago. Over millennia, as the size of our babies' brains grew and grew, we were forced to deliver them earlier and earlier, so their heads didn't get stuck. Some of these "preemies" died because their cries were just too weak to get their mom's attention when she was outside the cave cooking dinner. But some babies were born with the amazing new ability of screaming; sending an urgent *long-distance call* to their mom.

Why Are Babies Born with a Crying Reflex, but Not a Laughing Reflex?

Wouldn't it be fun if your baby was born laughing? There are two good reasons why he can cry up a storm, but it will take months before you get some real chuckles.

First, crying is easier than laughing. It takes less coordination, because it's one long sound made with each exhale. Laughter, on the other hand, is a series of rapid, short sounds strung together like pearls on a single breath.

Second, while laughter is a great way to flirt with your parents, crying is absolutely crucial for survival, from a baby's first minute of life. (That's why even premature babies are born with a crying reflex!)

Such brash, noisy babies may have attracted predators, but since their parents had fire and tools to fight them off that was probably not a big threat. On the other hand, this impressive blast effectively got the moms—and everyone else—instantly sprinting over.

We may never know exactly when human babies developed the gift of crying, but it's clear every person today is descended from babies who survived because they could "raise a ruckus." Your newborn's shrill cry is so powerful it can yank you out of a warm bed or hoist you off the toilet and get you shuffling over . . . with your pants at your ankles! (Not bad for a seven-pound weakling.)

But don't think of this crying as manipulation, or even as a request to get you to come. During the first few months, babies cry out of instinct, not out of intention. Your one-month-old has no idea he's sending you a message. His cries are like complaints he's muttering to himself, "Gosh, I'm hungry," or "Boy, I'm cold." But since you're right next to him, you're accidentally overhearing his conversation . . . with himself.

Within a few months, your baby will start to notice that crying

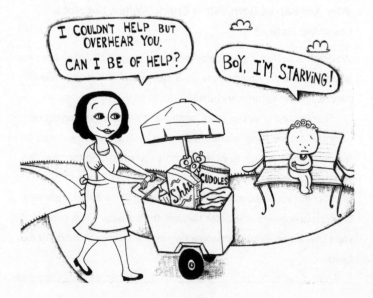

makes you hustle over. By four months, he'll have a little starter vocabulary of distinct coos, bleats, and yelps to communicate specific needs. (Around nine months, your infant may even start throwing out "phony" little shrieks just to get you to come play.)

You don't have to worry that responding to his cries might teach bad habits. Limit setting only becomes important after around nine months. But during the early months, you have a much more vital job: Building trust. Predictable, consistent, kind responses—*whenever he cries*—teaches your baby to have confidence in you and helps him grow up feeling loved and worthy of love! Psychologists call this great life foundation a secure *attachment*.

HOW A BABY'S CRY MAKES US FEEL

And, still Caroline cried, and Martha's nerves vibrated
in extraordinary response, as if the child were connected
to her flesh by innumerable invisible fibers.

Doris Lessing, *A Proper Marriage*

Babies have many built-in reflexes, and so do adults. Years ago, researchers proved that an infant's heart-shaped face, upturned nose, and big eyes give us the powerful urge to smile, kiss, and cuddle them for hours!

And we also feel compelled to urgently respond to a baby's wails. The sound of crying makes our nervous system snap into "red alert": The heart races, blood pressure throbs, palms sweat, and the stomach tightens like a fist.

Your baby's cry makes you want to help, and so do his actions. His little fists punching the air and his grimacing face can penetrate your heart like an arrow. (This powerful, biological impulse is exactly why it's so hard to wait outside the nursery while your baby cries himself to sleep.)

The good news is that young babies don't have the ability to be manipulative, rude, or critical. (Remember, they can barely burp without help!) Nevertheless, it's easy to take it personally and feel criticized when your baby screams and screams. His sobs can trigger feelings of helplessness, anxiety, and even a desire to run away. These wails may rekindle memories of past traumas, failures, humiliations, or insults. And, parents experiencing other stresses—such as fatigue, isolation, marital discord, financial stress, and so forth—are especially prone to feeling overwhelmed by crying. (See Appendix B for practical parenting tips for keeping your sanity these difficult days.)

Note: Anyone who has been in an airplane with a crying baby knows parents aren't the only ones who tune in to a baby's cries. Other adults, children, and even animals find the sound of a baby cry deeply upsetting and almost impossible to ignore. Check out the many cute viral videos of dogs singing and howling to calm fussy infants!

"TELL MOMMY WHAT'S THE MATTER": YOUR BABY'S THREE-WORD VOCABULARY

> *Our tiny baby's first word to us wasn't* Mama *or* Dada. *It sounded more like . . . well, a smoke alarm! She just blasted! It was scary because we had no idea exactly what she was trying to tell us.*
>
> Marty and Debbie, parents of two-week-old Sarah Rose

When you come home from the hospital, every fuss can sound like a problem and every cry an urgent alarm. But how can you tell exactly what your baby needs? Is your one-week-old's "I'm cold" cry different from his "I'm starving" wail?

Some experts claim they can tell a baby's need from the sound of his cries. That may be true after the first few months, but several studies show that's rarely the case earlier on.

A University of Connecticut study had moms listen to audio-taped yells from two different babies, a hungry one-month-old and a newborn who had just been circumcised. They were asked if the babies were hungry, sleepy, in pain, angry, startled, or wet. Only 25 percent identified the cry of the unfed baby as hunger (40 percent thought it was an overtired cry). Almost half called the cries of the circumcised baby a pain cry, but a third thought he was startled or angry.

Are experienced caretakers better at deciphering the cries? Finnish researchers asked eighty seasoned baby nurses to listen to recordings of babies. They were asked if a baby's sounds were wailing out of hunger or pain, a cry right after birth, or gurgling in pleasure. Surprisingly, even these pros only picked the correct cause 50 percent of the time—barely better than by chance alone.

By three months, your baby will make a rainbow of different utterances, from grunts to wails. However, during the first months, his compact brain simply doesn't have enough room to house a varied repertoire. He'll mostly make three simple sounds: whimper, cry, and shriek.

WHIMPER. This mild fussing sounds more like a request than a complaint. Think of it like a call from a neighbor asking to borrow some sugar. (Some have suggested that it is possible to distinguish between different whimpers, such as hunger, loneliness, and so forth. But that still remains to be proven.)

CRY. This good, strong yelp summons your attention, like when a kitchen timer goes off.

SHRIEK. Cries from any cause (hunger, cold, and so on) can escalate into shrieks—as shrill and disturbing as a smoke alarm—if they're not attended to.

Most of us would guess that whimpering means mild unhappiness; crying indicates more distress (such as being very hungry, thirsty, or cold); and shrieking signals an urgent problem (like pain). And we would be right, but only with a relatively easy child.

Fussy babies, those with naturally passionate or sensitive personalities, often lack the self-control to patiently proceed through their three-word vocabulary. Like little *rockets,* they skip the first two sounds and launch right into piercing wails. And, as with smoke alarms, it is impossible to tell—from the sound alone—if the problem is serious (a fire) . . . or minor (burned toast). And then their own screaming may make them so upset that it snowballs into even louder shrieking!

Another misconception is that crying is "the way" babies communicate. Fortunately, newborns also have a repertoire of gestures (cues) to help understand their needs. For example:

- Is your baby opening his mouth and rooting or putting his hand up to his lips? This could be a sign of early hunger.
- Is he rubbing his eyes, yawning, blinking, or staring out with glassy eyes? This usually means fatigue.
- Does he seem to intentionally look away from you or is he hiccupping? This could mean overstimulation.
- Is he grimacing, grunting, and trying to bear down? This could indicate the need to poop or simply that he feels food making its way through his intestines.

Fortunately, even a baby's most terrible shrieks are rarely danger signs. They're merely a show of a mild desire *plus* impatience. And your child will quiet as soon as he gets what he needs.

But what if the yelps persist even after a feeding, diaper change, and cuddle? What if you try everything and your poor little baby just keeps screaming? That's when the doctor will start to wonder if your baby has colic.

3

The Dreaded Colic:
A "CRYsis" for the Whole Family

• Colic means that a baby is crying for hours a day!
• Top five colic theories, from gas to acid reflux to parent anxiety.
• Colic clues: The ten universal facts about colic.

> *The sound of a crying baby is just about the most disturbing, demanding, shattering noise we can hear. In the baby's crying there is no future or past, only now. There is no appeasement, no negotiations possible, no reasonableness.*
>
> Sheila Kitzinger, *The Crying Baby*

Waaaa. . .waaaa. . .waaaaaa. . .WAAAAAAAAAAAAAAA!!!!!!!!
The word *infant* comes from Latin, meaning "without a voice." But colicky babies should really be called *mega-fants* or *rant-fants* because their wails are so loud!

Amazingly, tiny infants can shriek louder and longer than any adult. You would drop from exhaustion after five minutes of full-out screaming, but your tough little cutie can squawk for over an hour . . . with the tenacity of a prizefighter.

The word *colic* dates back to the ancient Greek word *kolikos,* meaning "large intestine or colon." That's because, back in Plato's time, parents believed crying was triggered by stomach cramps. Yet, as you'll soon learn, most babies with gas and noisy stomachs never make a peep. (More about this in chapter 4.)

HOW CAN YOU TELL IF YOUR BABY HAS COLIC?

The celebrated pediatrician Dr. T. Berry Brazelton asked 82 new moms to keep a three-month journal of their babies' fussy periods. Brazelton discovered that by four weeks, 50 percent of the babies fussed or cried more than two hours each day, and by six weeks, 25 percent fussed or cried more than three hours. A study of 2,700 newborns reported a daily average of two and a half hours of crying or fussing at around two months, with 10 to 20 percent vocalizing loudly more than three hours a day. Thankfully, by three months, few babies cried for more than an hour a day. (This pattern is why doctors used to call the problem the *three-months colic.*)

But how can you tell if your baby's crying is in the normal range or has crossed the line into colic?

A Connecticut doctor, Morris Wessel, studied that question and created a very precise definition for colic, the *Rule of Threes.* He stated that a baby has colic if he cries at least three hours a day, three days a week, for three weeks. (That's a lot of crying and doesn't even include the parents' crying!)

Today, the *Rule of Threes* is still mentioned in parenting books, but, honestly, it's totally unhelpful. Is a baby who wails for two hours

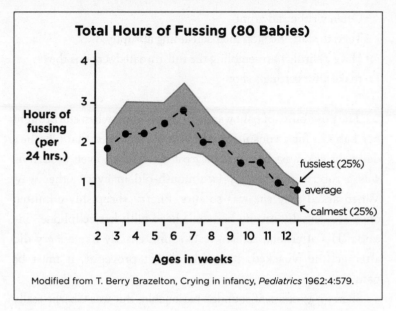

Total Hours of Fussing (80 Babies)

Modified from T. Berry Brazelton, Crying in infancy, *Pediatrics* 1962:4:579.

any less upset—or upsetting to his parents—than a three-hour wailer? So, in recent years, the whole three-hour cutoff has been tossed in the trash. Doctors have switched from using the term *colic* to describe these big-time fussers, to saying a baby has *persistent or inconsolable crying.*

Unfortunately, there's really no way to predict who will develop colic. No consistent association has been found between intense crying and a baby's gender, prematurity, type of milk, birth order, or a couple's age, income, or education. *Colic is truly an equal-opportunity parent nightmare!*

WHAT REALLY CAUSES COLIC?

Nine out of ten parents think their colicky infant is suffering from pain. And at first glance that seems to be a reasonable guess, since they:

- Often writhe and grunt
- Tend to start and stop their screaming abruptly
- Have a shrill cry resembling the full-throated screams they make after getting a shot

The possibility of pain was on Sherry's mind when she brought her baby in for a consultation. She was convinced that Charlie's daily shrieks must be a sign of great discomfort, even though he was a robust and healthy two-month-old in every other way. When asked why she was so sure, Sherry sheepishly admitted once accidentally hitting her son's head with her cellphone. She said, "His afternoon scream fests sound exactly like his cry did after getting whacked. I thought, 'That proves it, it must be pain.'"

Sherry's assessment sounded reasonable. But was Charlie really in pain, or had Sherry misread the situation?

Since prehistoric days, perplexed parents have tried to figure out why their babies suddenly erupt into screams. And they have come up with some doozies!

THE "EVIL EYE" (AND OTHER THEORIES): HOW OUR ANCESTORS EXPLAINED COLIC

> *Before I got married I had six theories about bringing up children; now I have six children and no theories.*
>
> John Wilmot, 2nd Earl of Rochester (1647–80)

Deciphering a Stone Age baby's cry may well have been the first multiple-choice question in human history!

Baby Krathnor is crying because:
    a. She's hungry.
    b. She's cold.

    c. She needs a fresh loincloth.

    d. A witch cast a magic spell on her.

Just one hundred years ago, people still believed that leeches could cure diseases and that babies were born blind. So, as you might imagine, some wild theories about why babies have prolonged crying have circulated for centuries.

The Top Five Ancient Theories of Colicky Crying

    1. Someone who hates the mom gave the baby the evil eye.

    2. The baby is possessed by the devil.

    3. Daytime is for adults to talk, and nighttime is the baby's turn.

    4. Crying is punishment for Adam and Eve's original sin.

    5. The mother's milk is bad (too thin, too thick, or filled with her angry emotions).

Even Shakespeare tossed in his two cents. In *King Lear* he proffered: *When we are born, we cry that we are come to this great stage of fools.* Babies are amazing, but I'm afraid the Bard was giving them a bit more credit than they deserve.

THE MYTH OF "BLOWING OFF STEAM"

> *Crying is good for the lungs the way bleeding is good for the veins!*
>
> Lee Salk

In modern times, parents and scientists have also made guesses about why some babies scream. Some even believe that fussing is a good thing. They say that babies—overexcited by the day's thrills—unwind by "blowing off steam." Others speculate that loud criers were more likely to survive during prehistoric times because they were fed more than their passive siblings.

But these ideas don't hold water:

- Colicky infants would have been *less* likely to survive during prehistoric times. Their screams might have attracted predators and enemies to their family's hiding place or enraged their primitive parents, leading to abandonment and infanticide.
- Screamers *do* eventually conk out from sheer exhaustion, but they're not little pressure cookers needing to "blow off steam." Letting a baby "cry it out" makes as little sense as letting your car alarm screech while you patiently wait for the battery to die.
- While some babies *do* get overwhelmed by the day's chaos, no normal baby should cry five-*plus* hours a day.
- The fact that fussy infants calm with car rides and soothing rhythms (sound, motion, sucking) is proof that they need help, not abandonment.

Note: PLEASE put your baby down if you feel yourself getting frustrated and angry. *Never, never shake your baby!* (Read more on the difference between safe, jiggly swinging and the violent jerks of shaken baby syndrome on pages 160–161.)

Letting your baby shriek to the point of exhaustion goes against all our parental instincts. And it can make your baby a little crazy! We get frustrated when our baby calms easily one day, but nothing works on another. Similarly, babies can get frustrated when their morning cry brings a reward of warm milk, but their nighttime cries are totally ignored.

Actually, the predictable repetition of your loving response is *the key* to building your baby's confidence. Quickly meeting your baby's *request* to be held or fed—dozens of times a day—strengthens her trust in you. Inconsistency creates insecurity.

You might then ask, "Is it ever okay to let my baby yell?"

During the first months, do your best to soothe upsets. If your two-year-old screams to hold the scissors and ignores your limit setting, you should lovingly acknowledge her desire (using the Toddler-ese technique described in *The Happiest Toddler on the Block*). But then, you may have to let her cry to teach her that when you say "No!" you mean it. Don't worry if you missed ten minutes of crying because you were in the shower. The mountain of love and cuddling you give throughout the day easily outweighs the occasional short-lived frustration. But teaching discipline to a two-month-old is way too early.

COLIC: THE FIVE MODERN THEORIES

Most doctors (and parenting books) suggest five possible triggers of inconsolable crying:

1. **TINY TUMMY TROUBLES:** Crying from digestive discomfort, such as gas, constipation, or cramps
2. **BIG TUMMY TROUBLES:** Crying from true intestinal pain, such as food sensitivity or allergy, excess "bad" bacteria, or stomach acid reflux
3. **MATERNAL ANXIETY:** Wailing triggered when babies sense their moms' fear and worry
4. **BRAIN IMMATURITY:** Crying from overstimulation in babies with extra-immature nervous systems
5. **CHALLENGING TEMPERAMENT:** An overreaction to minor upsets in infants with intense and/or sensitive temperaments.

Is one of these five the answer to this three-thousand-year-old puzzle? To arrive at the solution, like Sherlock Holmes, we need to follow the clues. When it comes to colic, there are ten key clues. And the true cause of colic must explain all ten.

COLIC: THE TEN UNIVERSAL CLUES

1. Colic starts around two weeks, peaks by eight weeks, and ends around three months.
2. Preemies get colic as often as full-term babies, but it never starts until their *due date.*
3. Colic cries come and go abruptly . . . and sound like the baby is in pain.
4. These grunts and screams often start during or just after a feeding.
5. Breast-fed babies have just as much colic as bottle-fed.
6. Colic tends to worsen in the evening: the so-called witching hour.
7. Colic is as likely with your fifth baby as with your first. It's unrelated to a parent's level of experience.
8. Colic often quiets—temporarily—with vigorous rocking, holding, and strong sound, such as from a car ride or a vacuum cleaner.
9. Colicky babies are healthy and happy between crying bouts.
10. In some cultures around the world, colic is rare or nonexistent.

Now, let's see if any of the five modern theories fits all ten clues and solves this ancient mystery!

4

~~~~

The Top Five Colic Theories, and Why They're (Mostly) Wrong

MAIN POINTS

- Do tiny tummy troubles (gas, constipation, or cramps) cause colic?
- Do big tummy troubles (food sensitivity or allergies, "bad" bacteria, lactose intolerance, or stomach acid reflux) cause colic?
- Does maternal anxiety trigger colic?
- Does a baby's brain immaturity lead to colic?
- Does a challenging temperament explain prolonged crying?

All five modern colic theories sound plausible, but let's follow the clues and see which—if any—makes it to the finish line.

THEORY 1: DO TINY TUMMY TROUBLES CAUSE COLIC?

All infants have gas! I'm sure you've witnessed your child's virtuoso performance of grunts, burps, and toots. For millennia, parents have had strong "gut feelings" that crying meant stomach discomfort. They were convinced that cramps, gas, and constipation caused colic, and they had two powerful allies in that thinking: grandmothers and doctors.

Does Gas Cause Crying, or Is That Just a Lot of Hot Air?

Experienced caregivers around the world have long recommended vigorous burping, tummy-massage and soothing teas for fussy babies. They've also advised nursing moms to avoid gassy foods. Doctors, too, have told moms to change their diets—or their children's formula—and to give medicinal drops to reduce intestinal gas.

But with all due respect, fussy babies don't have any more gas than calm ones. In 1954, Dr. Ronald Illingworth, England's top pediatrician, took stomach X-rays of normal and colicky babies. He found zero difference in the amount of swallowed air in the stomach. And studies on burp drops (simethicone) show them to be no more helpful at reducing crying *than plain water*.

Burping with the Best of Them

Babies don't cry from swallowed air. Nevertheless, they may gulp air during feedings and have more spitting up. Here's how to help your baby swallow less air and be a better burper:

1. Feed your baby sitting up. (Imagine how much air *you'd* swallow if you had to drink lying down!)
2. If your baby is a noisy eater, stop the meal—frequently—to burp.
3. Use a good burping position: Seat your baby on your lap, his chin resting comfortably in your cupped hand. Let him lean forward so he's doubled over a little. (I rarely burp babies over my shoulder, because the spit-up goes right down my back.)
4. Loosen the bubbles. Think of your baby's stomach like a glass

of soda, with little "bubblettes" stuck to the sides. Bounce him on your lap a few times and thump the back like a little tom-tom drum (ten to twenty times) to jiggle these free.

Poop Problems: Can Constipation Trigger Colic?

Babies pushing out poop look like they're struggling in a wrestling match. They often groan and twist, even when passing soft or runny stools. Fortunately, true constipation (hard poops) causes crying in very few formula-fed babies.

Why do babies grunt and strain so much if they aren't constipated? Think about it:

1. To poop, infants must tighten the stomach muscles and relax the anus . . . at the same exact moment. This is not easy to do. Many little babies just can't coordinate it and accidentally *clench* both at the same time and end up trying to force the poop out through a tightly closed anus.
2. Babies lay on their backs most of the time. Just think of how hard it would be for you to poop in that position.

Babies grunt and cry as they struggle to overcome these two challenges, not because they're in pain. (For more on infant constipation, see chapter 14.)

Is Your Baby Crying from the *Gastrocolic Reflex*?

Does your baby double up and complain a few minutes into a feeding? This twisting may look like indigestion, but it's probably just an overreaction to a normal part of digestion, called the *gastrocolic reflex* (literally, the *stomach-colon reflex*).

Your baby's digestive system is like a long conveyor belt. Food (milk) fills the stomach and then is slowly moved down through the long intestinal track as it is digested. Any leftover milk turns to poop, which gradually fills the lower intestine (colon).

At the next meal, the intestine needs to make room for a new load of food. So as the stomach fills, it sends an order to the colon to squeeze . . . and empty. (That's why babies often poop during or right after eating.)

Adults also have this reflex, although it's so mild that we're rarely aware when it's happening. Similarly, most infants take no notice of the reflex. But, for some infants, the squeezing feels weird and upsetting. The ultrasensitive babies who writhe and shriek after eating are usually the same ones who launch into screams when the phone rings or someone laughs too loud. You'll feel reassured that your baby isn't in pain when he calms quickly with the 5 S's.

Don't Soothe Crying Babies with Medicine

From the 1950s to the 1980s, doctors prescribed hundreds of millions of prescriptions of anti-cramp medicine for fussy babies. Bentyl was by far the most popular, but it also turned out to be one of the most dangerous. In 1985, doctors were horrified to discover that a number of babies receiving this "innocuous" antispasm drug suffered convulsions, coma, and even death.

Some Reasons Why Tiny Tummy Troubles Aren't the True Cause of Colic

> *It's not what we don't know that gets us into the most trouble, it's what we know . . . that just ain't so!*
>
> Josh Billings, *Everybody's Friend*, 1874

Despite the popularity of the idea that gas causes colic, the tiny tummy troubles theory can't be the basic cause of colic because it fails to explain these clues:

1. *Colic starts around two weeks, peaks by eight weeks, and ends around three months.*

   Yet, gas is present from birth (weeks before colic starts) and continues long past the time when colic ends.

2. *Preemies get colic as often as full-term babies, but it never starts until their due date.*

   Preemies have tons of gas. So if gas caused colic you'd expect them to cry on day one. Yet, preemies never get colic before their due date, which for many may not come until two to three months after birth.

3. *Colic tends to worsen in the evening: the so-called witching hour.*

   Babies have stomach rumblings twenty-four hours a day, so if gas or cramps caused colic the crying should happen at any hour, day or night.

4. *Colic often quiets—temporarily—with vigorous rocking, holding, and strong sound, such as from a car ride or a vacuum cleaner.*

   How could rocking, holding, or noise stop severe stomach pain?

5. *In some cultures around the world, colic is rare or nonexistent.*

   Babies around the world burp, toot, and poop. So if these caused colic, all cultures would have the same occurrence of persistent crying, but they don't.

THEORY 2: DO BIG TUMMY TROUBLES CAUSE COLIC?

Over the past thirty years, scientists have discovered several new causes of adult stomach pain. Four of these have been intensively investigated as possible colic triggers: food sensitivity (including allergies), an imbalance between good and bad intestinal bacteria, lactose intolerance, and stomach acid reflux.

Food Sensitivity and Allergies—"Un-Happy" Meals

If your breast-fed baby is fussy, you may have been told to stop eating spicy foods or avoid "gassy" veggies (broccoli, cabbage, and so forth). Garlic, onions, broccoli, and beans sometimes make *adults* gassy. But if they're so hard on a baby's stomach why is it that nursing moms in Mexico eat frijoles (beans) and moms in Korea munch kimchi (garlic-pickled cabbage) without their babies letting out a peep?

Studies show that what you eat flavors the womb fluid and breast milk, giving your baby a smorgasbord of tastes. That helps them get familiar with the foods they'll enjoy for the rest of their lives. So if you're a garlic lover, don't be surprised if your little one breast-feeds more heartily after you've had a plate of shrimp scampi!

Fussy infants rarely improve when foods are eliminated. Nevertheless, if your breast-fed baby is very fussy, it's reasonable to skip some *problem foods* for a few days to see if the wailing winds down. (The key offenders are citrus, strawberries, tomatoes, beans, cabbage, broccoli, cauliflower, Brussels sprouts, peppers, onion, and garlic.)

Unlike food sensitivities, allergies are an overreaction of the immune system as it tries to protect us from foreign proteins. In older kids and adults, the fight between your body and cat dander or pollen typically takes place up high, causing a runny nose and sneezing. But with infants, the usual allergy battleground is in the intestines.

As just mentioned, allergies are triggered by *proteins*. And, for babies, the main foreign proteins come from milk. For decades, we've know that babies can react to proteins in cow's milk and soy formulas. These molecules zip through the intestinal wall into the baby's blood stream like flies passing through a torn screen door. Once in the blood they can provoke allergic reactions. (For the first year or two of life, the intestinal walls are immature—especially leaky—and allow molecules through more easily.)

But what about nursing? Can a baby be allergic to his mom's milk? In 1983, Swedish scientists proved that colicky breast-feeders are never sensitive to their mom's milk, however they can be allergic to proteins that sneak from the mom's intestine into her bloodstream and then into her milk. Within minutes of a mom eating a meal, tiny bits of the proteins make it all the way from her belly to her breast! Proteins entering the breast milk usually peak eight to twelve hours after a meal.

Babies with food allergies suffer many bothersome symptoms, from severe crying to rashes, nasal congestion, wheezing, vomiting, and diarrhea (often laced with strings of bloody mucus).

Fortunately, most infants tolerate all the yummy proteins in our diet. The fact that colic is as common with breast-fed babies as those receiving formula—even though the latter take in *tons* more cow's milk protein—argues against food sensitivity or allergy being a common cause.

Having said that, the most common baby food allergies are to cow's milk (the majority of all baby allergies) and soy (10 percent of milk allergic babies are soy allergic, too). Rare causes of baby allergies are eggs, nuts, and shellfish. (It should come as no surprise that some babies have trouble with cow's milk. After all, this food is lovingly made for baby *calves,* not for our hungry *babies.*)

If your baby is fussy, before you decide to switch formula or go on a chicken and water diet, skip ahead and see if you can soothe your baby's upsets with the 5 S's.

Note: Blood in your baby's diaper will raise your heart rate, but it's usually no more worrisome than having a little bloody mucus come from your nose when you have nasal allergies. Nevertheless, contact the doctor any time you see blood in the stool.

Stimulant Food: Is Your Baby on a Caffeine Jag?

Some of us can sleep right after downing a double espresso, while others toss and turn after a bite of dark chocolate! So it's no surprise that some breast-fed babies are fine when their moms drink coffee, while others get hyper after their moms have caffeine (coffee, tea, sodas, energy drinks, dark chocolate, and so forth) or stimulant medicine (diet pills, nutritional supplements, decongestants, Chinese herbs, and the like). Caffeine collects in breast milk for four to six hours after it is consumed.

Studies haven't shown an increase in upsets among babies whose moms drink coffee before nursing; nevertheless, if your baby gets restless and fussy a few hours after you have caffeine, avoid it for a few days to see if the fussing improves.

"Bad" Bacteria: Is Colic a Form of Germ Warfare?

For centuries, people have celebrated the health benefits of cultured foods, like yogurt. It turns out that these foods contain "good" bacteria (probiotics), which help keep us healthy. These important microbes make vitamins, aid in our digestion, and—like an army of microscopic vigilantes—they patrol our intestines keeping bad bacteria at bay.

An amazing thing about breast milk is that it naturally boosts the probiotics in a baby's intestine. In fact, one of the *best* of these good bacteria has the name *Lactobacillus acidophilus*, which literally means the "milk bacteria that loves acid." Large amounts of *L. acidophilus* in the intestine of breast-feeders is a big reason why their poop is much less stinky than that of formula feeders.

Several studies have reported that "good" bacteria can prevent serious intestinal problems, including colic. These reports have led to an explosion of consumer products, such as probiotic-filled drops, powders, and formulas.

Unfortunately, other studies cast doubt that these little germs are the long-sought cure for colic. A review of a dozen studies found that colic relief from probiotics was no better than a coin toss: In six it helped; in six it flopped. An Australian study found zero benefit from probiotics, regardless of whether the colicky babies were breast- or bottle-fed.

Probiotics are definitely not the "silver bullet" they've been touted to be. Nevertheless, they may reduce intestinal inflammation in some babies; and that might lessen cramping from an overactive *gastrocolic reflex* (see page 35). So, *if* the 5 S's don't help, ask your doctor if she thinks probiotics may be useful.

Lactose Intolerance: Another Wrong Idea

Lactose literally means "milk sugar." It is made in the breast by linking together two other sugars (glucose and galactose). Lactose is so abundant in mama's milk that it actually makes the milk sticky!

Unlike regular table sugar (sucrose) or high-fructose corn syrup, lactose is very good for infants because it improves health three different ways:

- It's digested into glucose, the key fuel for your baby's body . . . and brain.
- It provides loads of galactose, essential for building your baby's nervous system.
- Any excess lactose that passes through the intestine undigested gets fermented—to gas plus a vinegar-like acid—in the lower intestine. This causes frothy, acidic stools that can irritate your baby's skin (not so nice). But the mild acid can also save your baby's life by killing bad bacteria and boosting *Lactobacillus acidophilus* (fantastic).

The lactose your baby eats is digested by the enzyme *lactase* in the intestine. With age, adults have less and less lactase. This makes some of us *lactose intolerant,* causing bloating, bellyache, and diarrhea after eating dairy products. This adult problem led some doctors to speculate that colicky babies might be suffering from stomach pain from lactose intolerance. Soon the markets were flooded with lactose-free formulas (soy, lactose-free cow's milk, and special hypoallergenic milk) and special lactase-containing colic drops . . . all claiming to be a *cure* for colic. But this multimillion-dollar promotion was based on hype not health. A Canadian study showed no improvement from lactose-free formula in colicky babies. And an Australian study found no reduction in crying when fussy infants were given lactase in their mother's milk.

Stomach Acid Reflux: Do Babies Cry from Heartburn?

For many years, pediatricians have wondered if colic might actually be a burning pain caused by acid squirting back up the wrong way from the stomach (also known as gastroesophageal reflux, or GER). One book even trumpeted it as "the cause of all colic." But hundreds of millions of dollars spent on baby antacid medicine (and big-pharma ad campaigns) have been wasted. It's now proven that GER *rarely* causes colic.

Australian doctors examined twenty-four babies who were so irritable they had to be hospitalized (all under three months of age). Each was checked for acid reflux, but only one had it. In fact, studies now show that even babies who *do* have severe reflux usually have no pain. Out of 219 babies hospitalized because of severe reflux, 33 percent had excessive vomiting and 30 percent were failing to gain weight, but few had just excessive crying.

A University of Pittsburgh study confirmed that acid reflux medicine makes no difference for most babies with colic. Doctors caring for 162 infants with marked crying after eating gave half the babies a powerful antacid; the rest got a placebo. What happened? Fifty percent of babies got better on the medicine . . . *but* 50 percent got better on the placebo, too.

In truth, *all* babies have reflux; we just call it by a different name: *spitting up*. There is a muscle at the bottom of the esophagus that keeps stomach juice from flowing back up to the mouth. For the first six months it is pretty weak, so babies often burp up a smidge of their last meal . . . mixed with a bit of stomach acid. And, some barf huge amounts, with no crying at all. Doctors call them *happy spitters* and suggest just burping them better and not overfeeding. For these families, the biggest problem caused by reflux are milk stains on clothes and sofas.

Despite years of mounting evidence, 82 percent of pediatricians are still fooled into overprescribing acid suppression medicines. (Most of these medicines are not even FDA approved for infants under one year of age.) Frustrated doctors try to calm frustrated parents by giving out hundreds of thousands of antacid prescriptions every year.

Not only is this medicine unnecessary, it may be harmful! Stomach acid is an early line of defense against the bacteria your baby sucks off her fingers and lips and swallows every day. Studies show that antacid drugs allow bad bacteria to grow in the stomach and may raise the risk for pneumonia and gastroenteritis. And one type of antacid even had to be pulled from the market because it was found to cause sudden death.

When should you suspect that your baby has a reflux problem? Only if you see these telltale signs:

- She vomits more than five times a day and more than an ounce each time.
- Her crying occurs with most meals—even early in the day.
- The crying jags don't improve after three months of age. (Acid reflux doesn't lessen until infants reach four to six months of age . . . well after colic is gone.)
- She has episodes of hoarseness or wheezing.

Note: So, even if your baby has improved on acid reflux medicine . . . ask your doctor about trying her off it for a few days, to see if the medicine is really necessary.

Big Tummy Troubles Strike Out as the Main Cause of Colic

Today, medical experts estimate that only 5 to 10 percent of colic is due to major gastrointestinal problems. Most of these are due to food sensitivities or allergies, very few from acid reflux or bacterial imbalance, and virtually none from lactose intolerance. Indeed, the big tummy troubles theory fails to explain several of the colic clues:

1. *Colic starts around two weeks, peaks by eight weeks, and ends around three months.*

   If allergies, bad bacteria, lactose intolerance, or acid pain caused crying, the screams wouldn't disappear after three months . . . because older infants still get tons of milk, their intestines are *still* loaded with regular, non-probiotic bacteria, like *E. coli,* and they still have plenty of spitting up . . . yet most colic is totally gone by then.

2. *Preemies get colic as often as full-term babies, but it never starts until their due date.*

   Preemies are constantly exposed to milk protein and lactose, they have tons of smelly bad bacteria in their intestines, and spit up daily. So, if those problems caused crying they should have colic long before their due date.

3. *Colic tends to worsen in the evening, the so-called witching hour.*

   Protein and lactose consumption, intestinal bacteria, and acid reflux are the same morning and night. So there would be no witching hour if they caused colic.

4. *Colic quiets—temporarily—with vigorous rocking, holding, and strong sound, such as from a car ride or a vacuum cleaner.*

How would a car ride soothe inflamed intestines or heart-burn? Indeed, rocking and pressure might even squirt more acid up from the stomach, worsening reflux pain. And a vacuum cleaner sound certainly can't affect a baby's intestinal bacteria or ability to digest lactose.

5. *In some cultures around the world, colic is rare or nonexistent.*
   Yet all babies around the world eat lots of lactose, spit up frequently, and have tons of *E. coli* and other stinky bacteria in their stools.

THEORY 3: DOES MATERNAL ANXIETY CAUSE COLIC?

Any mom who has felt fear and anxiety surrounding the birth of her new baby might wonder if these could affect her newborn. That was Trina's big concern.

With her ruby lips and lush, black hair, Tatiana was exquisite. But her delicate form was balanced by a strong temperament. She had her parents' passionate personalities, and Trina and Mirko could not have been more thrilled. But as the weeks went by they wilted as Tatiana's feistiness turned into shriekathons.

Trina called her doctor after one particularly bad afternoon. She confided, "I'm a very sensitive and intuitive person. Is it possible that Tatiana is, too? I know she's only four weeks old, but could she be picking up on all the stress that I'm feeling?"

Trina said that after the baby's birth she'd had terrible pain from her C-section and just days later they lost most of their possessions from a flood in their apartment.

"The nest we created for our baby collapsed like a house of cards and we had to move into our friend's living room. When Tatiana developed colic at three weeks, I thought her screams might be from all the anxiety she felt from me."

The birth of a healthy infant is a glorious experience, but it's a rare mom or dad who doesn't have episodes of anxiety and self-doubt. New parents can feel overwhelmed for so many reasons:

- Caring for the baby is harder than they expected. They *thought* they were prepared, but the exhaustion and 24/7 demands hits them like a ton of bricks.
- They have little baby experience. In the past, new parents cared for the babies of friends and relatives all during their childhood. Today, most new moms have little hands-on experience. As amazing as it sounds, modern parents are probably the least experienced in human history!
- They feel like everybody is butting in. New parents get constant advice, even from total strangers. "Pick her up!" "Don't pick her up!" "Feed on demand!" "Feed on a schedule!" Being peppered by all these can whittle down your confidence and magnify doubts.
- They have little help: Don't think that having a nanny is "cush" . . . *it's the bare minimum.* Just because you're the mom doesn't mean you must do everything on your own: calm crying, juggle feeding, handle all chores, and so forth. Until one hundred years ago, most new moms had help every day from several baby-savvy adults!

A New Mom's Feelings of Inadequacy

Aye, aye, aaaaaye! Am I really ready for this?

Unless you've spent lots of time babysitting or helping with younger siblings, mothering is neither automatic nor instinctive. For most of us, caring for a baby is the toughest job we've ever had. So don't be surprised to sometimes find yourself wishing you had six arms—like a Hindu goddess.

Here are the top ten stresses that make new parents struggle:

1. Intense fatigue
2. Inexperience
3. Isolation from family and friends
4. Intrusive family and friends
5. Inconsolable crying (the baby's, that is)
6. Irritating arguments with your spouse
7. Instant loss of job income and gratification
8. Insecurity about your body
9. Intense pain (from delivery or breast-feeding)
10. Indelible barf stains on every piece of clothing you own

As you become a mom, you enter a vulnerable psychological space. Being in the midst of one of life's most intense experiences—particularly having a colicky baby—can increase your vulnerability to other life stresses. The sum effect is that many women suffer from distorted self-perceptions and waves of anxiety and depression. (For more on postpartum depression, see Appendix B.)

Fortunately, once the early pressures pass, most parents melt into a warm love that is often more powerful and profound than any they have ever felt before.

So, please be patient and tolerant with your baby, your partner, and, especially with yourself!

Anxious Mama Is Not the Answer

Colicky infants are born, not made.

Dr. Martin Stein, *Encounters with Children*

Persistent fussing can cast a shadow over your confidence and make you wonder if your fear or frustration is causing at least some of the crying. But babies are just babies! It may feel like your feelings are written on your forehead in lipstick (Sad! Mad! Nervous!), but your baby is just too immature to read your complex emotions.

Note: Your newborn's hand trembling, chin quivering, and startling at loud noises are not signs of nervousness. These are caused by your baby's immature nervous system and disappear within a few months.

Nevertheless, there are a few ways a mom's anxiety could nudge her baby into crying:

• Anxiety can reduce breast-milk supply or block letdown, thus frustrating a hungry baby.
• Distraught moms may be too distracted and emotionally unavailable to comfort their crying infants.
• Anxious moms may lack the confidence to swaddle, shush, and swing the baby as emphatically as needed to calm the screaming. (See the discussion about vigor in chapter 7.)
• Nervous moms impatiently jump from one calming method to another, never doing any of them fully and successfully.

The nervous-mom theory fails to explain three key colic clues:

1. *Colic starts around two weeks, peaks by eight weeks, and ends around three months.*

   Parents are most anxious during the first days of a baby's life. So, if worry caused colic, you'd expect fussing to peak right after birth.

2. *Preemies get colic as often as full-term babies, but it never starts until their due date.*

   These fragile babies can turn even secure parents into nervous wrecks. So if anxiety provoked colic, you'd expect premature babies to suffer crying jags from the first days and weeks after birth.

3. *Colic is as likely to occur with your fifth baby as with your first.*

Experienced moms are way more confident, so if anxiety led to colic, you'd expect a woman's fifth baby to be much less colic prone than her first, but the risk doesn't vary with birth order.

Trina didn't need to worry! Her stress hadn't burdened Tatiana's tender psyche. In reality, the opposite is usually the case. Our babies' wailing triggers a red alert in our nervous system, making *us* tense and anxious . . . not vice versa!

THEORY 4: COULD A BABY'S IMMATURE BRAIN CAUSE COLIC?

Young infants have the coordination of drunken sailors and the mental speed of, well, babies. Could colic be triggered when a baby's immature brain gets overstimulated by the avalanche of new sights, sounds, and smells they encounter? It's a popular theory because, let's face it, newborn brains are so undeveloped. But let's look at exactly what is immature in there and see whether that might lead to hours of wailing.

Brain Skills Your Baby Was Born With

Imagine you're going on a long trip but can only bring one small suitcase. What essentials would you pack? In a way, that's your baby's dilemma. As he prepares for birth, there's *no way* he can stuff all the skills of a three-month-old into a head that's small enough to fit through your ten-centimeter cervix.

So babies have to narrow their list and "pack" only the skills that are vitally needed to survive outside the womb.

What essentials would *you* choose for your baby to pack? Walking? Smiling? Saying "I love you, Mommy"? Over eons, Mother Nature picked five indispensable abilities to squeeze into a baby's apple-size brain:

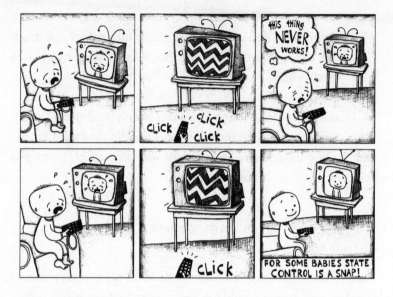

1. Life-support systems: Used to maintain blood pressure, breathing, and so forth.
2. Reflexes: Dozens of automatic behaviors, such as the ability to sneeze, suck, swallow, and cry.
3. Five senses: The ability to touch, taste, see, smell, and hear opens the door to the surrounding world.
4. Muscle control: Limited abilities to reach out, lift the head, and imitate your face as the baby learns to interact.
5. State control: A special ability to turn attention on (to watch and learn) and off (to recover and sleep).

Of all of these abilities, state control is the one most related to colic.

State Control: Babies Tune In to the World . . . or Shut It Out

Can your baby sleep when the TV is blasting? When fussing starts, does it always escalate, or can he sometimes calm all by himself? These are signs of *state control*.

This type of "state" has nothing to do with whether you live in Ohio or Florida. It describes the six levels of a baby's alertness: deep sleep, light sleep, drowsy, quiet alert, fussy, and screaming. (Smack in the middle of this rainbow of arousal your baby's face will peacefully relax as he surveys the sights around him. That's the magical state called *quiet alert*.)

One of the first jobs of your baby's brain is *state control* (to stay calm for a period or have a nice, long sleep). Like a TV remote, state control lets your infant "keep the channel on" when something's interesting or "shut the TV off" when it's time for bed.

Infants with better state control are good at self-soothing: shifting easily from crying to calm. When the world gets too wild, they protect themselves from the craziness by shifting attention: 1) staring into space; 2) sucking their own lip or finger; 3) retreating into sleep; or 4) gazing away from the commotion, as if to say, "This is *soooo* exciting, I just have to look away to catch my breath!"

After the first weeks, your baby will spend increasing amounts of time alert as he starts "waking up" to all the amazing sights and sounds in your home. However, paying more attention can overexcite him and overwhelm his state control. He may become so engaged by the circus around him that he'll watch until he's totally fatigued. Even then, he may resist surrendering to sleep, staring out bug-eyed and exhausted.

If your little one gets locked into screaming, part 2 of this book will show you how 5 S's can rescue him during the meltdown.

"Help! . . . I'm Stuck in a Closet!" Can *Under*stimulation Cause Crying?

> *Your baby is not crying to make you pick him up, but because you put him down in the first place.*
>
> Penelope Leach, *Your Baby and Child*

Newborns can get overloaded by the parade of new sights, sounds, and smells around them. Some experts have even suggested that fussy babies need the isolation of a quiet, dark room to help them recover. But is stillness really best for fussy babies?

Our image of the perfect nursery is one where infants sleep in total quiet, but the flat, unmoving bed and stony silence feels as strange to your baby as being placed in a dark closet would feel for you.

As strange as it sounds, your baby doesn't want—or need—peace and quiet. Babies love monotonous repetition. (They don't even get bored drinking milk for every meal, for six months.)

On the contrary, too much stillness drives babies more nuts than overstimulation. The *absence* of monotonous repetition—the hypnotizing rhythms they enjoyed before birth—is hard for them to tolerate. (It takes a few months for state control to become strong enough to handle long days without hours of calming, rhythmic reassurance.)

The bottom line is that both *under*- and *over*stimulation can upset your child . . . and the worst is experiencing both. Babies subjected to the daily chaos of life—in the absence of calming rhythms—are easily driven past their tolerance point.

Is Immaturity the Long-Sought Cause of Colic? Close, but No Cigar!

Brain immaturity is a big piece of the colic puzzle. But it fails to explain two key clues:

1. *Preemies are no more likely to have colic than full-term babies.*

   If brain immaturity caused screaming, preemies—*with their super-immature brains*—would definitely be the fussiest of all babies!

2. *In some cultures around the world, colic is rare or nonexistent.* Infants in other cultures don't have more mature brains than babies in our culture. So the absence of colic in some cultures proves that brain immaturity can't be the main basis of persistent crying.

THEORY 5: DOES CHALLENGING TEMPERAMENT CAUSE COLIC?

Are challenging kids the product of poor parenting? Or, are some babies just natural-born screamers?

Nature or Nurture: What Sets Your Baby's Personality?

Did you hear the one about the boy who had all F's on his report card? He handed it to his dad, lowered his head, and asked, "Father, do you think my problem is due to heredity . . . or my upbringing?"

A thousand years ago, people believed the temperament of babies was the result of the milk they were fed. Ancient experts warned never to feed a baby milk from a donkey or from a wet nurse with a weak mind, poor scruples, or from a crazy family.

Today it's widely accepted that about 50 percent of our personality traits are genetic hand-me-downs from our parents. So it's no surprise that shy parents tend to have shy kids and passionate parents often give birth to little chili peppers.

Andrea was the baby of Zoran, a former race-car driver, and Yelena, a psychiatrist with a high-pressure practice. Fussy from the very first days, Andrea had escalated to shrieking out her complaints almost twenty-four hours a day by the time she reached two months. Zoran laughingly noted, "She's as tough as nails, but what else would you expect? Two Dobermans don't give birth to a cocker spaniel!"

Temperament: The Sea Your Child Sails On

People are wrong when they think that quiet babies are good and fussy babies are bad. In truth, some gracious, softhearted babies are fussers because they can't handle the turbulence of the world around them.

Renée, mother of Marie-Claire, Esmé, and Didier

Think of your baby like a boat and her temperament as the sea she sails on. Infants with a stable boat (good self-calming ability) on a smooth sea (a calm temperament) sail easily through the first year. But unstable boats (poor self-calming ability) or rocky seas (challenging temperament) make babies prone to being pushed into crying by the day's tumult of sensations.

Luckily, most babies are mild tempered.

Easy-Tempered Babies: A Walk in the Park

Mellow from the first days of life, these babies register their complaints with mild fussing, as if to say, "Please, Mummy, it's a teensy bit too bright in here!"

These little "surfer dudes" have no trouble taking the craziness of the world in stride.

However, babies who are sensitive or intense—or, heaven help you, both—often launch into screaming outbursts, like boats tossed in a storm.

Challenging Temperament: Little Babies with Big Personalities

Lizzy and her twin Jennifer were like peas in a pod, both supersensitive to noise and sudden jolts. When unhappy, they cried with deafening force. Their one difference: Jenny could eventu-

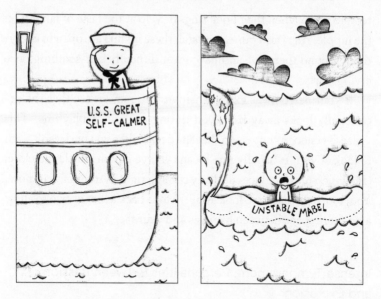

ally quiet her own upsets, but once Lizzy's screams got rolling, she had no ability to rein herself in.

Infants like Lizzy are tough because their personalities are too big for them to handle. They're often given funny nicknames by parents who are trying to laugh—rather than cry—during the difficult early days and nights. Amanda's parents christened her "Demanda," Charlotte's mom called her "Gassy Gussy," and Lachlan's parents dubbed him "General Fuss-ter."

Two types of temperament are particularly challenging: babies who are sensitive to everything . . . and those who are super-passionate and intense.

Sensitive Temperament: Perceptive Infants as Fragile as Crystal

Do you have extra-sensitive friends or relatives who get annoyed by sounds, messy rooms or strong smells? Similarly, sensitive newborns tend to jump when the phone rings or yelp at the taste of lanolin on the nipple. Alert and pure as crystal, these infants are open to everything around them . . . and have great difficulty self-soothing once crying starts.

If your newborn is extra-sensitive, you may notice that she occasionally looks away from you during feeding or playtime. This "gaze aversion" is not a sign that she doesn't like you or doesn't want to look at you. It usually just means you've gotten a little too close. (Imagine a ten-foot face suddenly coming right in front of your nose. You, too, might need to look away!) Move back a foot or two to allow a bit more space between her eyes and your face.

Intense Temperament: Personalities Between Passion . . . and Explosion

All babies experience flashes of frustration. Calm kids take these in stride, but intense babies tend to explode. It's as if the "sparks" of everyday distress fall onto the "dynamite" of their volatile temperaments . . . and *Kapow!* And, once these babies are wailing, stopping the upset may be hard, even when they get what they seem to want.

Jackie witnessed this intense crying when her passionate two-month-old got hungry.

Jeffrey would announce his hunger by letting out a "Feed me or I'm gonna die!" shriek and I would leap off the sofa, pulling my breast out as I ran to him. But he'd often ignore my dripping boob at his mouth and continue to cry, shaking his head from side to side as if he were blind!

I worried that he might think of my breast as a hand trying to silence him rather than my loving attempt to rescue him. Despite his protests, I persisted until he could latch on. And then, lo and behold, he'd eat as if I hadn't fed him for months.

Jackie smartly realized that Jeffrey wasn't intentionally ignoring her gift; he was just an itty-bitty baby . . . dealing with a great big personality.

What's *Your* Baby's Temperament?

Even on the first days of life, you may get glimpses of your baby's budding temperament. These questions may help you better understand his personality on a scale from placid to peppery:

1. Do sudden little shocks (such as bright lights or cold air) trigger a slight whimper or full-out scream?
2. When you lay him on his back, do his arms usually rest serenely or flail about?
3. Does he startle easily at loud noises and sudden movements?
4. When hungry, does he slowly increase his fussing or accelerate right into wailing?
5. When he's eating, is he like a little wine taster (calmly taking sips) or a passionate, gulping *all-you-can-eat* eater?
6. How hard is it for you to get his attention when he's in a vigorous cry? And how long does it take to get him to settle back down?

These won't perfectly predict lifelong temperament, but they definitely begin to shed light on your child's uniqueness.

Does a Baby's Temperament Last a Lifetime?

As babies grow up, they don't get less intense or sensitive, but they do develop skills to help balance their temperamental swings. By three months, your baby's smiling, cooing, rolling, grabbing, and chewing will help her handle excitement and annoyance. And another month or two after that she'll add the superb self-soothing skills of laughter, mouthing objects, and moving about.

With time, the excitement that used to ignite her shrieks will start a bubbly flow of giggles. So if you have a challenging baby, don't lose heart. Passionate infants often become the biggest laughers and most talkative members of the family. ("Hey, Mom, look! Look! It's incredible!") And sensitive infants often grow into the most compassionate and perceptive children. ("No, Mom, it's not purple. It's lavender.")

Goodness of Fit

A good part of temperament is inherited, but just as brown-eyed parents may wind up with a blue-eyed child, mellow parents occasionally give birth to a *T. rex* baby who makes them want to run for the hills!

It's a challenge caring for a baby whose temperament differs dramatically from our own. We may handle a sensitive baby too roughly or an intense baby too gently. But part of our job as parents is to try to figure out our baby's personality and nurture him the way that suits him the best.

Is Temperament the Cause of Colic? Probably Not

Sensitive and passionate overreactions definitely play a role in colic. But challenging temperament can't be the root cause of crying because it fails to explain three key clues:

1. *Colic starts around two weeks, peaks around six weeks, and ends by three to four months.*

   Since temperament lasts a lifetime, a challenging temperament should make colic persist—or even worsen—after the fourth month of life.

2. *Preemies get colic as often as full-term babies, but it never starts until their due date.*

   One would expect immature preemies with sensitive or intense personalities to get even *more* overwhelmed and have more severe colic than mature, full-term babies. Also, one would expect the crying to start right away, not weeks or months later.

3. *In some cultures around the world, colic is rare or nonexistent.*

   All cultures have babies with intense and passionate personalities. If temperament caused colic, all cultures would have super-fussy babies.

So, what *does* cause persistent crying? As you'll see in the next chapter, the theory that best explains the mystery of colic is the missing fourth trimester.

5

The True Cause of Colic:
The Missing Fourth Trimester

MAIN POINTS

- The first three trimesters: Your baby's happy life in the womb.
- The great eviction: Why babies are so immature at birth.
- Why your baby wants (and needs) a fourth trimester.
- The missing fourth trimester: The true cause of colic.

So if the root cause of colic isn't stomach troubles, anxiety, immaturity, or inborn temperament . . . what the heck makes babies so upset?

Do you know the story of the blind men and the elephant?

Once upon a time, there lived four blind men in a village. One day, they heard the children shouting, "There's an *elephant* in the village!" Having no idea what an elephant was, the blind men wanted to understand what all the excitement was about, and they asked to be guided up to the beast for a turn examining it.

After running his hands over a tusk, the first to approach the beast said, "An elephant is a long, curved thing, like a spear!" The next, clutching the leg, shouted, "Not at all! This thing is thick and upright—it feels just like a tree." As they argued, the third touched the ear and compared it to a giant leaf. Finally, the last blind man, wrapped up in the elephant's trunk, declared triumphantly that they were all wrong—the animal was like a big, fat snake.

Each was so sure his view was the whole truth that he didn't consider the possibility that he was getting only part of the picture.

Centuries of wise men and women trying to explain colic have focused only on bits of the truth. Some heard a baby grunting and thought gas was the problem. Others saw a grimace and thought it was pain, or noted that cuddling helped and assumed the baby was manipulative. However, like the elephant, the cause of colic only becomes clear when all the clues are woven into one single concept: the missing fourth trimester.

The First Three Trimesters: Your Baby's Happy Life in the Womb

It's logical to think your fetus is ready to be born after nine months of pregnancy. God knows *you* are ready! But babies really need a little more time. The nine months—three trimesters—in the womb are a time of unbelievably complex development, but during the first months after birth, babies are still very immature and benefit from generous amounts of womb-like rocking, shushing, cuddling, and care until they are mature enough to smile, coo, flirt, suck their fingers, and become a full partner in the *mommy and me* relationship.

Newborns love the soothing sensations they enjoyed in the womb. But doing these correctly requires knowing what the world was like inside there.

Let's travel back in time—and into your womb—to imagine life as your baby experienced it. Do you see the muscular walls and silky membranes wafting in the tropical amniotic waters? Over there is your pulsating placenta. Like a twenty-four-hour diner, it serves up a continuous feast of food and oxygen. And in the seat of honor—protected from hunger, germs, cold winds, mean animals, and rambunctious siblings—is your precious baby. Part astronaut, part merman, he floats weightlessly in the warm fluid.

For nine months, he has developed at lightning speed. His body has grown a billion times in weight and infinitely in complexity. Even now, his brain contains 100 billion nerve cells! (About as many neurons as there are stars in the Milky Way.) And he is creating millions of new neural connections every second!

Let's zoom in on his last month of fetal life. It's really tight in there. Like a little yogi, he's folded like a pretzel. But contrary to popular myth, his cozy quarters are neither still . . . nor quiet. It's jiggly and noisy! Your baby bounces with your every step (imagine when you hustle down the stairs or attend an exercise class). And

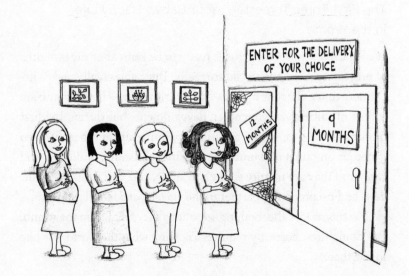

blood whooshing through the placental arteries creates a rhythmic din that's louder than a vacuum cleaner.

Amazingly, all this commotion doesn't upset your fetus. In fact, he finds it soothing. (That's why many unborn babies stay calm all day long, but get restless as soon as their mom lies down for the night.)

But if life is so ideal in there, why do we give birth after just nine months? After all, other animals, such as elephants and whales, happily carry their babies for eighteen to twenty-two months.

The Great Eviction

Upon thee I was cast out from the womb.

Psalms 22:10

Mama horses keep their babies inside until they've gotten strong enough to run . . . on the first day of life! They grow as big as they can . . . yet still be small enough to slip out.

In the very distant past, our ancestors had small-headed babies who were kept in the womb until their bodies were strong and mature. (Newborn chimps, for example, can tightly cling to their mom's fur as she hurries through the forest.) But super-smart brains increasingly became our babies' ticket to survival, and over millennia pregnant moms stuffed more and more new skills into their unborn babies' brains, filling them like Christmas stockings. Eventually the heads got so big they began to get stuck during birth . . . killing both themselves and their mothers!

The tight confines of the birth canal would have ended the advancement of our big brains, but for four evolutionary changes that allowed fetal brains to keep growing:

1. **SLEEK HEAD DESIGN:** Babies developed slippery skin, squishable ears, and tiny chins and noses to keep their big heads

from getting wedged. (During the first years of life, your baby's tiny chin will grow fast and catch up to the size of the rest of his face.) The head developed a mushable skull that could elongate into an easy-to-deliver bullet shape as it went down the birth canal.

2. **HEAD ROTATION:** If you want to get a tight ring off a finger or a cork out of a bottle, *twist* it as you pull. Similarly, our babies' big heads rotate as they pass through the snug birth canal to keep them from getting stuck.

3. **NO-FRILLS BRAINS:** Over time, the tightly packed brains of our babies had to start eliminating bits and elements that weren't absolutely needed during the first weeks of life. For example, your baby's brain leaves out much of the cerebellum (the balance/coordination center) and most of the brain's *insulation*. (Like wires, our nerve cells are insulated, but newborns—missing much of that—have frequent twitches and startles . . . like little short circuits.)

4. **EVICTION:** Big-brained babies who were *booted out* while they were still immature were less likely to get stuck in the birth canal.

With each passing generation, big-brained babies grew up into smarter moms who figured out new and better ways to protect their evicted little babies, such as warm clothing and sling-like carriers to give them the soothing sensations of the womb.

Today, even with these changes, giving birth is still a tight squeeze. As you probably know, the dilated cervix measures ten centimeters. Unfortunately, a baby's head is eleven and a half centimeters across. No wonder midwives call the birth canal the *ring of fire* and we refer to giving birth as *labor*.

Note: Childbirth has always been a heroic act, and, until recently, it put both baby and mother in mortal peril. The Aztecs greatly honored women who died giving birth. They believed these mothers entered the highest level of heaven, alongside warriors killed in battle.

Big-Brained Babies

Imagine giving birth to a three-foot-long, eighty-pound newborn. Of course, delivering a baby half the height or weight of an adult would be ridiculous. Now, imagine giving birth to a baby with a head half the size of an adult's. That sounds even more absurd, but the fact is that such a head would be *small* for a newborn! A new baby's noggin is almost *two-thirds* as big as an adult head. (Ouch!) But, fortunately, it is also stream-lined, elongated, and slippery.

Your Baby Needs a Fourth Trimester

> *The baby, assailed by eyes, ears, nose, skin, and intestines at once, feels it all as one great blooming, buzzing confusion.*
>
> William James, *The Principles of Psychology,* 1890

A fourth trimester of cuddling is the birthday present your baby really wants!

You may think your peaceful nursery offers your new baby the perfect environment, but from her point of view your home feels like it's part wild Las Vegas casino . . . and part dark closet!

After birth, a baby's senses are bombarded by new experiences. From the outside world comes a jumbled assault of lights, colors, and textures. From the inside come powerful new feelings such as gas, hunger, and thirst. Yet, alternating with all this is the distressingly *under*stimulating stillness of the room. (Imagine how strange your nursery must seem after the loud, quadraphonic shushing of your womb.)

Mabel, the mother of four daughters, piqued my curiosity when she mentioned she believed colic was caused by *electricity*! She said, "I noticed my kids are more stimulated and struggle to fall asleep when the house is brightly lit in the evening. I think the long "daytime" we artificially create with electric lights tricks them into thinking it's still "time to play." Our kids consistently sleep better when we dim the lights at night or use candles."

Over the first couple of weeks, your infant will deal with all these changes by "shutting down" and sleeping a lot. But as she wakes up to the world, she may get overwhelmed (by both the chaos *and* unnatural stillness), unless you hold, rock, and suckle her for long chunks of the day. Those sensations duplicate the womb and trigger the powerful calming reflex.

A "Womb with a View": A Parent's Experience of the Fourth Trimester

> *When the baby comes out, the true umbilical cord is cut forever . . . yet the baby is still, in that second, a fetus . . . just a fetus one second older.*
>
> Peter Farb, *Humankind*

The first time you see and touch your new baby is utterly unforgettable. His open gaze and downy skin will capture your heart. But newborns can also make us feel intimidated. They seem so vulnerable with their floppy necks, funny breathing, and tiny tremors.

You and your immature baby are now united by a virtual umbilical cord—your ears and his cry—his sharp yelps yanking you back to your little one's side.

"When Stuart came out he didn't seem ready to be in the world," said Mary. "He required constant holding and rocking to keep him content. My husband, Phil, and I joked that he was like a squishy cupcake needing to go back in the oven for a little more baking."

Mary and Phil realized that Stuart needed a few more months of "womb service." But it's not easy being a walking uterus! Doing everything your uterus did—holding, feeding, nurturing your baby—takes all day long, and you may find yourself still in your pj's at five P.M.! (Try not to get too self-critical if the house is a mess, emails go unanswered, and dirty dishes pile up.)

Yet, as hard as you're working, your baby thinks that being in your arms for *just* twelve hours a day is a rip-off! If your baby could talk, he'd say, with pouty disdain, "What are you complaining about? You used to hold me twenty-four hours a day and feed me every single second!"

Strangely, many parents have been brainwashed into believing that their babies must immediately learn to be independent. They treat children more like they are brains they must train, rather than gentle spirits needing to be nurtured.

Other cultures see infants very differently. In Bali, babies never sleep alone and barely leave the arms of an adult for the first four months. On the 105th day, they conduct a holy ceremony to welcome the baby as a new member of the human race. The infant is given his first sip of water, and an egg is rubbed on his arms and legs to give him vitality and strength. Only then are his feet finally allowed to touch Mother Earth.

It's no coincidence that in cultures such as Bali, where colic is extremely rare, parents naturally give babies a fourth-trimester experience.

The Great American Myth: Young Babies Can Be Spoiled

Hide not thine ear to my cry.

Lamentations 3:56

We all know two things about unruly children:

1. There are lots of spoiled kids out there.
2. You don't want your child to become one of them.

But will being too attentive to your newborn's cries make him manipulative?

Fortunately, the answer to that question is "Hell no!"

A century ago, parents were cautioned not to mollycoddle their babies for fear of turning them into undisciplined little nuisances. A 1914 pamphlet from the U.S. Children's Bureau sternly warned moms not to accidentally teach their children that crying will get them what they want, lest an infant become "a spoiled, fussy baby, and a household tyrant whose continual demands make a slave of a mother."

It's easy to feel manipulated when your baby screams every time you lower him into the crib. But, remember, at birth you abruptly robbed your child of his daily feast of rocking, holding, and rhythmic sound. One mom joked, "No wonder they cry. Like a detox program, we make our new babies go *cold turkey* from the 24/7 snuggling they had in the womb!"

Fortunately, it's impossible to spoil a baby during the first four months of life. Native American parents have traditionally held their babies all day and suckled them all night. And those babies grew up to be brave, respectful, and self-sufficient. Ignoring your baby's cries is as unlikely to make him independent as leaving him in dirty diapers will toughen his skin.

In 1972, Johns Hopkins researchers Sylvia Bell and Mary Ainsworth found that meeting an infant's needs quickly and tenderly during the early months made him more poised, patient, and trusting when tested at one year of age. Bell and Ainsworth's work became the basis of a new area of understanding of *attachment*.

Attachment psychology teaches that a rapid, loving response to a baby's cries is the very foundation of strong family values. When your arms cuddle your baby, or warm milk satisfies him, you're telling him, "Don't worry. I'll always be there when you need me." This builds your baby's trust and becomes the solid basis for deep friendships and successful intimacy for the rest of his life.

As the Bible says, "To everything there is a season." Around nine months is the earliest time you should think about spoiling. Before that, nurturing your baby's confidence is one hundred times more important than pushing him to be independent.

Note: After nine months, many more situations will arise when you'll want to teach patience and impulse control. "I know you want to hold my knife, sweetheart. But it's dangerous! See . . . danger! Sharp! Ouch! Ouch!!" (For tips on teaching respect and discipline to tots from eight months to five years of age take a look at *The Happiest Toddler on the Block* book/DVD.)

THE MISSING FOURTH TRIMESTER: THE TRUE BASIS OF COLIC

> *There's no place like home.*
>
> Dorothy, *The Wizard of Oz*

After centuries of myths and confusion, it is now clear that the true basis of colic is when babies are deprived of the calming rhythms of the womb.

You might ask, "If the missing fourth trimester makes babies cry, why don't they all get colic?" The reason is simple: Most babies have mild temperaments and good self-calming abilities, which help them

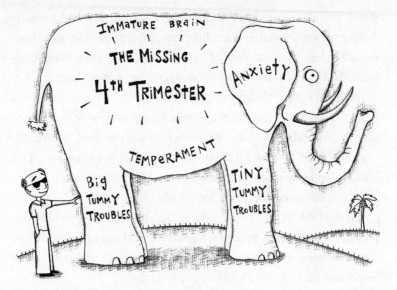

handle being born too soon. Despite all the overstimulation and understimulation, they're able to soothe themselves. On the other hand, babies with challenging temperaments or poor state control dramatically overreact to the same experiences. These infants desperately need soothing womb sensations to turn on the calming reflex.

Note: For the science lovers, here is an equation that I think best explains the factors that trigger colic:

$$\text{Colic} = \frac{[\text{Overstimulation} + \text{Total Stillness}] - \text{Rhythmic Calming}}{\text{Temperament} + \text{Brain Maturity}}$$

Babies with easy temperaments and great state control can handle the amazing new world around them. But infants with challenging temperaments and poor self-calming ability get pushed into colic by too much excitement, too much stillness, and too little womb rhythms. That's why many babies can be rescued from colic with a fourth trimester filled with the calming help of the *5 S's*.

Looking back at the five modern colic theories, you can see how tummy troubles (such as gas, the *gastrocolic reflex*, or food allergies) might push a baby with an intense temperament "over the edge." And how mild discomforts might trigger huge meltdowns in babies with poor self-calming state control.

Putting the Fourth Trimester Theory to the Test

There's a reason behind everything in nature.

Aristotle

Does the missing fourth trimester solve the three-thousand-year mystery of colic and explain all ten colic clues. Let's see:

1. *Colic starts around two weeks, peaks by eight weeks, and ends around three months.*

   The fourth trimester perfectly fits this clue.

   Initially, newborns sleep so much they rarely get over- or under-stimulated. After two weeks, though, babies start staying awake for longer periods. Mellow babies easily handle this increased alertness and the over- and under-stimulation it brings, but sensitive or intense babies and poor self-calmers begin to get overwhelmed. That's why persistent crying starts at around that time.

   By six weeks, alert babies can turn into major screamers if they are subjected to excess chaos and too few calming rhythms. (No wonder screaming peaks at that age.) By four months, all babies are better at self-calming (such as cooing, observing, laughing, sucking fingers, and turning away when too excited). At last, your little one is mature enough to stay serene with less holding, rocking, and shushing. Now he's ready to be born!

2. *Preemies get colic as often as full-term babies, but it never starts until their due date.*

Preemies tend to be calm, even in noisy intensive care units. They're not so great at focusing their attention, but their immature brains are skilled at staying asleep. With less alert time, preemies tend not to get overstimulated. They don't "wake up" until they get close to their due date . . . which is when their colic usually begins.

3. *Colic cries come and go abruptly . . . and sound like the baby is in pain.*

Colicky cries sound identical to the wails babies make when they're in pain. But fussy babies are usually just over-reacting to trivial experiences (loud noises, burps, and so forth). They're like smoke alarms that sound a major alert, when the only problem is a bit of burnt toast.

The fact that so many shrieky crying bouts quiet with car rides; strong, white noise; or suckling at the breast makes it obvious that these babies are not in pain.

4. *These grunts and screams often start during or just after a feeding.*

Babies who cry during or right after a meal are usually just overreacting to their *gastrocolic reflex* (the intestinal squeezing that occurs when the stomach fills with food and the colon starts pushing the poop toward the anus). Most babies have no problem with this reflex, but at the end of the day (and the end of your baby's patience), this intestinal sensation may be the last straw that launches him into hysterics.

The *gastrocolic reflex* lasts our entire life, but after four months it no longer triggers crying because as babies age they become much better at self-calming, even in the face of over- or under-stimulation.

5. *Breast-fed babies have just as much colic as bottle-fed.*

Breast-feeding doesn't change the balance of over- and under-stimulation. And it doesn't alter a baby's temperament or boost state control. That's why breast- and bottle-fed babies have the same chances of developing colic . . . and equally benefit from calming fourth trimester rhythms.

6. *Colic tends to worsen in the evening: the so-called witching hour.*

   Just as some toddlers crumble at the end of their birthday parties, babies can unravel after a day's mix of tumult and stillness. By evening, vulnerable infants start to bubble like pots of hot pudding unless they're given soothing fourth trimester sensations.

7. *Colic is as likely with your fifth baby as with your first. It's unrelated to a parent's level of experience.*

   Your first four babies may stay calm—despite lots of excitement and silence—while your fifth has an intense temperament and poor state control that makes him fall apart without lots of holding and rocking.

8. *Colic often quiets—temporarily—with vigorous rocking, holding, and strong sound, such as from a car ride or a vacuum cleaner.*

   Since each of these tricks imitates the womb, this clue is compelling proof that colic is caused by a missing fourth trimester. After four months, there is less need for the calming help of these old friends.

9. *Colicky babies are healthy and happy between crying bouts.*

   If the main reason for colic is trouble dealing with over- and understimulation, it makes total sense for these fussers to be healthy and happy until they're pushed over the edge.

10. *In some cultures around the world, colic is rare or nonexistent.*

    The babies of Botswana bushmen, for example, rarely—if ever—suffer from colic. These moms. hold their infants almost twenty-four hours a day, nurse them frequently, and constantly rock and jiggle them. In essence, they mimic the womb for months.

I hope I've begun to persuade you that the missing fourth trimester is the only explanation that really fits the ten colic clues. Yet, make no mistake about it, impersonating the womb can totally fail when done incorrectly.

In part 2, you'll learn everything you need to know to perfectly imitate your womb . . . to soothe crying fast *and* boost your baby's sleep.

PART TWO

The Ancient Art of Soothing a Baby

6

~~~

The Fourth Trimester:
The Woman Who Mistook
Her Baby for a Horse

MAIN POINTS

- Your baby is not a horse!
- The developmental leap from four days to four months of age is huge.
- Ancient lessons from moms whose babies don't get colic.

> *That which was done is that which shall be done; and there is no new thing under the sun.*
>
> Ecclesiastes 1:9

YOUR BABY IS NOT A HORSE

Imagine, it's a crisp spring day, gleaming like a jewel. Yesterday your life changed with the birth of a beautiful baby boy. This morning, as the nurse wheels his bassinet into your room, your tiny son turns his head to you . . . and flashes a huge grin! Then he vaults out of his bed

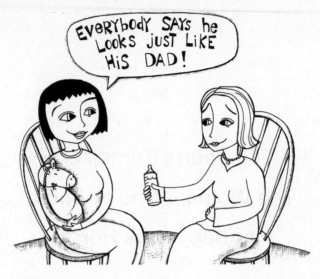

into your arms and—with a laugh that makes your heart melt—chirps, "You're the best mom in the whole, wide world!"

Wow! That would be fun. But, of course, it's totally sci-fi. Human babies are vulnerable and immature when they enter the world. But some animal babies *are* super-talented . . . from the very first day of life.

Newborn horses, for example, can run on day one. It's a simple question of survival. A baby horse will perish if it is not powerful enough to gallop away from hungry wolves. That's why colts have such big, strong bodies. During birth, their chest and shoulders are often a tight fit, but they have absolutely no trouble sliding out their sleek heads.

Our babies, on the other hand, survive because of their big, strong brains. Their smushy little bodies squirt right out, but their heads . . . well, that's another story. At birth, a baby's head is already a pretty hefty melon. And over the next three months, it balloons another 20 percent in size!

Like watching a caterpillar turn into a butterfly, witnessing your infant's transformation from a soft little newborn into a smiling, engaging member of the family, as the fourth trimester draws to a close, is beautiful and awe inspiring.

THE SURPRISING TRUTH: THE LEAP FROM FOUR DAYS TO FOUR MONTHS

> *When Audrey was two months old, she peed on me, then suddenly smiled. I know it sounds crazy but I was ecstatic!*
>
> Debra, mother of Audrey and Sophia

At prenatal classes, I often ask pregnant couples to list the differences between four-day-old babies and four-month-olds. Many of the first timers think it's a silly question and laughingly say, "Ha! Not much! They're all little babies." But the experienced parents usually pipe up and say, "Oh my God, you have no idea!"

Newborns are beautiful, but their abilities are quite limited. Four-day-olds can barely coo or turn their head to see who's speak-

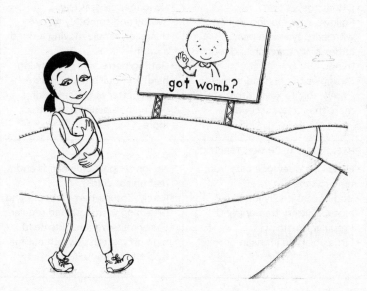

Four-Day-Olds	Four-Month-Olds
SENSORY ABILITIES	
• Focuses on faces 8 to 12 inches away • Loves looking at red things and light/dark designs • Begins to recognize your scent and the sound of your voice • Easily focuses on people across a room	• Quickly turns head to see you or find out where a voice is coming from • Easily recognizes your face and starts noticing when someone is a stranger
SOCIAL ABILITIES	
• Watches you talking with interest, but doesn't try to participate • Attracted to sounds (voices, shush, etc.) • Stares at faces or close objects • Struggles to imitate your facial expressions (such as sticking out your tongue) • Calmly looks around empty room	• Waits for you to stop talking before taking a turn cooing • Prefers human voices, especially yours • Face brightens when you enter the room • Gives a huge grin when you smile • Likes company, gets upset when ignored
MOTOR ABILITIES	
• Often crosses eyes • Follows slow-moving objects with jerky eye movements • Little ability to reach and touch things • Struggles to get hand to mouth (rarely able to keep it there for more than a few seconds)	• No longer crosses eyes • Swiftly and smoothly follows things or people moving around a room • Getting better aim (may swing hand and pull off your glasses!) • Much better at finger sucking, sometimes lasting a minute or more
PHYSIOLOGICAL CHARACTERISTICS	
• Hands and feet look blue from time to time • Body occasionally jolted by hiccups, jittery tremors, and irregular breathing • Little ability to lift head or roll	• No longer gets blue hands and feet unless cold • Rarely hiccups, never tremors, and breathing is smooth and regular • Easily rolls over and lifts head high off mattress (watch out for falls off the bed!)

ing. By contrast, four-month-olds' delicious smiles and glowing eyes reach out like a personal invitation to share some fun.

Months and months may pass in our lives without a whole lot of change. But during the first four months of life your baby will make amazing leaps in development.

These extraordinary weeks will speed by faster than you can possibly imagine . . . and they will never return. So enjoy cuddling and carrying your sweet little newborn as you give her the serenity and security of a last few months of womb-like pleasure.

Cuddling Builds Brains

A study done at Canada's McGill University asked "Does extra cuddling make animals smarter?" The researchers looked at two groups of baby rats. The first group had "loving" moms who generously licked and stroked their pups. The second group received much less affection.

When the rats became old enough to learn mazes and puzzles, scientists noticed that the cuddled animals were extra-smart. They had developed an abundance of connections in a part of the brain crucially important (in rats and people) for learning.

Bottom line: Cuddling feels good, and may boost a baby's brain development.

OUT WITH THE *NEW*, IN WITH THE *OLD:* THE ANCIENT WISDOM OF THE FOURTH TRIMESTER

Remember how Luke Skywalker triumphed by using the forgotten powers of the Jedi? Well, over the past fifty years, our society has discovered that many serious problems can be answered by returning to the great wisdom of the past, such as practicing yoga, mind-

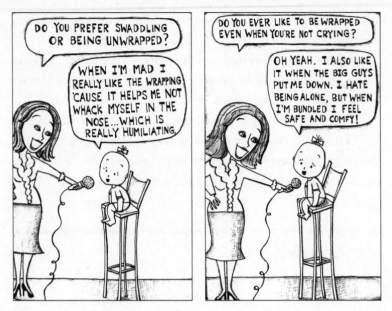

fulness, exercising, following a paleo diet, recycling, and eating organic.

Some people think the past holds little value, but our basic biology is profoundly linked to ancient times . . . and that is especially true with babies.

It may sound odd, but in most respects, our infants are probably very similar to infants living thirty thousand years ago. We can't go back in time to check, but by studying so-called primitive tribes, we can do some virtual "time travel" to get a better idea of how prehistoric moms may have soothed their young 'uns.

Note: Please don't be fooled by the word *primitive*. It may conjure up images of backward cultures, but these peoples live in complex societies and possess wisdom of which we are quite ignorant, such as the medicinal power of rare plants, how to find water in the desert . . . and even how to prevent colic!

PAST PERFECT: LESSONS FROM THE !KUNG SAN

For thousands of years, the !Kung San (or African bushmen) lived in isolation on the plains of the Kalahari Desert. Over the past fifty years, however, the !Kung have graciously allowed scientists to study their lives, including how they care for babies.

These reports are particularly interesting, because !Kung infants hardly ever cry.

!Kung infants have as many fussy periods as our babies, but their parents are so skilled that their fussy bouts average only sixteen seconds. More than 90 percent of the time their wails end in under a minute.

!Kung infants may lack material possessions, but by comparison, many of *our* babies lack a key *maternal* possession—long hours of being carried and cuddled. Careful examination of these African moms reveals three things underpinning their stunning success:

- They hold their babies almost twenty-four hours a day.
- They breast-feed around the clock.
- They immediately respond to their babies' cries, usually within ten seconds.

The !Kung carry their babies in leather slings all day and sleep with them all night. Their close proximity allows them to respond to any fussiness with quick little nursings—up to one hundred times a day. Does all this "indulgence" spoil their babies? Nope. Despite the lavish and immediate attention, !Kung kids grow up happy and exceedingly self-sufficient.

SCIENCE AND THE FOURTH TRIMESTER: RESEARCH POINTS THE WAY . . . BACK

Imitating the womb to calm colic isn't the only ancient wisdom that the Western world has ignored for centuries. Over the past sixty years, researchers have rescued another prehistoric skill from the brink of extinction: breast-feeding.

Within days of your baby's birth, her sucking makes your milk magically start to flow. This sweet, nutritious, easy-to-digest food is exactly what the doctor, and the baby, ordered. It gives a steady stream of nutrition, similar to what she enjoyed in the womb.

In the early 1900s, many moms in our culture lost confidence in their milk. After millions of years of being developed to perfection, breast milk was pushed aside by mass-produced artificial formula. The new "milk" was promoted as equally healthful—and more hygienic. Doctors jumped on the formula bandwagon, convinced that milk from a chemist was better than milk from the breast.

Increasingly, new moms sought medicine to dry up their breasts. By the 1950s, the few women who tried to breast-feed often failed because they had no experience and little professional guidance. By the 1960s, breast-feeding had become so rare that women who did it were considered radical, eccentric, or backward!

As unbelievable as it sounds, within two generations, our culture almost lost a key ability that had sustained our species for millions of years. Fortunately, many committed women (and men) were appalled by this trend. Through their great efforts, groups such as La Leche League were launched, and specialists were trained to revive this wonderful skill.

In recent decades, breast-feeding has rebounded, spurred by an avalanche of research on its special benefits. I'm thankful we have formulas for babies who are unable to nurse. But all groups agree, if you can do it, "breast is best" for babies.

Studies show that breast milk helps boost immunity, protects against obesity, reduces SIDS, and even lowers a woman's risk of breast and ovarian cancer. Today, even formula companies recommend women breast-feed before they switch to their products.

7

The Key to Happy Babies:

The Calming Reflex

and the *5 S's*

- Newborns have many great built-in behaviors and skills called reflexes.
- The calming reflex: Your baby's natural *off switch* for crying.
- The 5 S's: How to mimic the womb to turn on the calming reflex.

Once, while caring for a very fussy baby, I had the fantasy that, under one arm, I found a *secret button* to instantly turn off the tears. I know it sounds crazy, but it appears that babies *do* have a kind of "reset button" to soothe most crying.

Learning to master this "off switch" is easier once you undertand how baby reflexes work. (If you already have a very fussy baby, feel free to skip to chapter 8 for immediate help and come back to this chapter once things are under control.)

REFLEXES: BRILLIANT THINGS YOUR BABY CAN DO AUTOMATICALLY

Imagine trying to teach your baby how to suck or poop. Thankfully, you don't have to because newborns have about seventy automatic behaviors—reflexes—tucked into their jam-packed brains. The great thing about reflexes is that they don't have to be learned or practiced. Like blinking and coughing, reflexes are built-in. Many are so important they're even present from day one of life . . . and before!

All reflexes are:

- reliable: Every time a doctor hits your knee to test your reflex, your foot jumps out. It can be done a hundred times in a row and almost always works.
- automatic: Reflexes can be triggered without you even thinking about them. Some even work while you sleep.
- turned on by specific triggers and thresholds: Okay, this sounds technical, but it just means that reflexes only get flipped on by specific actions, and only when the trigger is strong enough. In other words, whack the knee *exactly* right and you'll have 100 percent success getting a knee reflex. But hit it an inch too high or tap it too gently (below the threshold), and you'll have 100 percent failure.

Most of your baby's reflexes are there to keep her safe and well fed during the early months. The rest are either *fetal* reflexes (important only before birth) or *leftover* reflexes (neurological versions of the appendix, probably very useful to our ancient ancestors, but of no value today).

You'll have fun catching your baby showing off these amazing tricks. Here are some to watch for:

1. **SAFETY REFLEXES:** Preventing injury, sometimes for our entire lives.

   Crying. This is the mother of all baby safety reflexes! Triggered by any sudden distress, it's also perfectly tuned to launch *your* nervous system into action and get your heart—and feet—racing to help.

   Sneezing. We often think of these as a sign of a cold, but baby sneezes are usually just little noses trying to eject bits of dust and mucus.

2. **FEEDING REFLEXES:** From the moment of birth, these help your baby consume life-sustaining milk.

   Rooting. Touch your baby's cheek near the lips (or right on the lips) and his mouth will turn toward the touch, open, and then shut. Rooting helps your baby locate and grasp your nipple . . . even in the dark. Don't worry if you stroke the cheek and your baby doesn't respond. Rooting is a *smart* reflex: It only turns on when an infant is hungry. If you touch his cheek and nothing happens, he's probably not needing a meal yet.

   Sucking and swallowing. Do you have ultrasound photos of your little cutie sucking his thumb before birth? After your baby roots and latches onto the nipple, sucking and swallowing get flipped on to send the milk down to the stomach.

3. **FETAL AND LEFTOVER REFLEXES:** These responses either help before birth or are unimportant ancient leftovers.

   Stepping. Hold your baby under the armpits (slightly leaning forward) and let the soles of his feet touch the floor. A few times out of ten, you'll see one leg suddenly straighten and the other bend. (Try leaning your baby a little to one side so one foot has more pressure under it than the other.) During the last months of pregnancy stepping may allow babies to shift position and prevent pressure sores.

   Grasp. Press your finger into your baby's palm or the sole of his foot, and he'll usually grab on with his fingers or toes. This may seem like a trivial little parlor trick, but it's actually critically important . . . for baby *apes*. Newborn chimps have to be able to cling to their mom's fur while she's scurrying through the jungle. (Be careful. Your baby's iron grip can yank off your glasses or pull a handful of "fur" from Daddy's chest!)

Moro. This is the famous "I'm falling" reflex. It flips on when a baby gets startled (by a jolt, loud noise, or her head suddenly falling back). The Moro reflex causes your baby's arms to shoot open, then come together in a big hug, as if she's trying to grab hold of you. It has probably saved countless baby monkeys whose moms were able to catch their outstretched arms as they started to fall.

As your baby matures, these clunky old reflexes will be retired and forgotten, like a toddler's tattered old blankie. But early in life his responses are literally lifesaving.

In addition to these, there's one more precious reflex that all babies have: the calming reflex. (It was first described in *The Happiest Baby* in 2002.)

THE CALMING REFLEX: NATURE'S OFF SWITCH FOR BABY CRYING

As our ancestors moved into villages, they needed to walk much less, and so their babies spent less time being carried and jiggled. Deprived of these sensations, babies started getting fussier. For hundreds of years, parents misread this crying as a sign that their fragile new babies were overstimulated.

These moms mistakenly believed that their fussy babies needed more gentle rocking and softer songs. Those loving acts are great for keeping calm babies calm, but to soothe screaming babies need *jiggly* motion and *strong* sound.

Remember, reflexes require actions to be done vigorously enough to exceed the threshold. Flipping on the calming reflex requires the jiggle and loud shush of the womb.

Interestingly, the calming reflex isn't there to soothe upset *infants;* it probably evolved to calm *fussy fetuses!*

Fetuses who wiggle around too much can move into a breech position and get stuck as they start coming down the birth canal. This can kill both the baby and the mom! How brilliant of Mother Nature to make the natural sensations of the womb put babies into a mini-trance the last two months of pregnancy to keep them from moving into risky positions.

Like most newborn reflexes, the calming reflex fades around four months after birth. But, thankfully, a little hint of it remains with us for the rest of our lives, which is why we're soothed by womb-like ocean sounds, rocking in a hammock, and being cuddled. In older infants, children, and adults, these sensations work as learned expectations, not automatic reflexes. Older children and adults certainly *enjoy* holding and rocking, but babies truly *need them.* And fussy babies need them desperately.

So if your baby continues to yell himself hoarse even after feeding, burping, and a diaper change, try soothing him this "old" new way.

Ten Ways to Impersonate Your Uterus

Clever parents have invented dozens of ways to lead distraught babies from wails to serenity. Here are ten of the best:

1. Holding
2. Dancing
3. Rocking
4. Swinging
5. Swaddling

6. Feeding

7. White noise

8. Singing

9. Pacifiers

10. Smart sleepers

Parents have used many of these for millennia, but our generation is the first in history to know that they work by switching on the calming reflex. Most soothing techniques fall into one of five categories: swaddling (snug holding), side/stomach position, shushing (white noise), swinging (motion), and sucking . . . the 5 S's. (A smart sleeper is a newly developed infant bed that intelligently responds to infant fussing with just the right amount of motion and sound—that any particular baby needs—to turn on the calming reflex. It can soothe middle-of-the-night crying and dramatically boost sleep.)

THE 5 S'S: TURNING ON YOUR BABY'S CALMING REFLEX

> *There should be a law requiring that the* 5 S's *be stamped onto every infant ID band in the hospital. For our frantic baby, they worked in seconds!*
>
> Nancy, mother of two-month-old Natalie

In the early 1900s, baby experts told mothers to respond to strong crying by: 1) feeding, 2) burping, 3) giving a dry diaper, and 4) checking for an open safety pin. When those didn't settle the screams, parents were told that their babies had colic and nothing could stop the crying for the next three months.

Amazingly, a century later, some doctors still give the same advice. (Moms from cultures around the world would *never* accept the idea that it's normal for babies to fuss or cry many hours a day!)

If you have a frantic newborn, the *nothing-to-do-but-wait* advice is intolerable. Few impulses are as powerful as the desire to calm our crying baby. Yet, while the desire to quiet crying is an instinct, knowing how to do it is not; it's a skill. Luckily, it's a skill that's pretty easy to learn.

Peter is a high-powered attorney and the father of Ted and Emily. When his kids were born, Peter and his wife, Judy, had little baby experience. So after the birth of each child, I reviewed the fourth trimester and 5 S's with them. Much later, Peter wrote:

> It has been more than ten years since I learned the 5 S's. Yet I remember them perfectly and I love teaching them to my friends! I love to see their amazed looks when a large, lumbering male—like me—collects their distraught baby and quickly calms the crying.

These five simple techniques give new moms and dads a great sense of accomplishment.

1st *S*: Swaddling—A Feeling of Pure "WRAPture"

Snug swaddling is the cornerstone of calming: the essential first step in soothing your baby and keeping him happy. That's why traditional cultures from Tbilisi to Timbuktu swaddle to keep their babies happy.

Wrapping imitates the continuous touch and snug cuddling of the womb. Of course, skin-to-skin contact is also great for soothing babies. But when it doesn't stop the fussing, swaddling can work wonders.

Fussy babies often fight the wrapping and cry even harder. But don't be fooled into thinking that the struggling means your little one wants or needs his hands free . . . nothing could be further from the truth. Crying babies strain against the blanket because they just can't stop their arms from flailing. If left unwrapped, their arms windmill, thrash and startle . . . making them even *more* upset.

Interestingly, swaddling alone doesn't always calm the crying, but by reducing the flailing you'll help your baby notice the next *S's you do*, which *will* flip on the reflex.

2nd *S*: Side/Stomach—Your Baby's Feel-Good Position

Most infants are perfectly happy to lie on their backs. But once upset, the back position can set off the Moro reflex (see page 88) and give your baby a panicky feeling of falling, which can turn startles into thrashing and screams.

Fortunately, rolling your baby to the stomach or side (facing down a little) can stimulate a womb-like sensation in the inner ear (the balance center). For some babies, this is so effective that it's all they need to *turn on* the calming switch.

Note: The back is the *only* safe position for sleep. But unfortunately, it's the *worst* position for comforting a frantic baby.

3rd *S*: Shushing—Your Baby's Favorite Soothing Sound

Strong, harsh shushing is music to your baby's ears. It mimics the whooshing he heard from the blood rushing through the placenta and uterus. This loud rumble continuously surrounded your fetus for all nine months.

It's a little counterintuitive to use intense white noise with babies, but they love that sound because it's a powerful trigger for the calming reflex.

For many babies, white noise is the key to fourth trimester calming. And the louder the cry, the louder the shush needs to be for effective soothing. (That's why so many parenting books recommend using vacuum cleaners and hair dryers to shorten bouts of screaming.)

In a rush to get out of the house, Marjan put off feeding her hungry baby for a few minutes to finish getting ready for work. Two-week-old Bebe didn't care much for this plan and wailed impatiently for food. Two minutes after Marjan entered the bathroom to dry her hair, Bebe suddenly quieted. Marjan panicked; was her tiny baby okay? She threw open the bathroom door and was relieved to see that her daughter was totally fine. Bebe had stilled the instant Marjan turned on the hair dryer.

Marjan shared her great discovery with her parents, but they were not supportive. They thought it was dangerous to use such a loud sound to calm an infant: "It's so loud it will make her go crazy!"

Despite their concerns, Marjan used her new "trick" with 100 percent success to soothe Bebe's crying. (But only when her parents weren't around.)

4th S: Swinging—Moving in Rhythm with Your Baby

Womb-like motion is one of the top baby-calming tips used by parents all around the world. Lying on a flat, motionless bed may appeal to us, but many babies hate it. Like a sailor coming to land after nine months at a sea, your baby may hate the stillness of your home after nine months of constant jiggling.

Note: To stop screams, the motion may need to be a bit vigorous at first (fast, tiny jiggles . . . no more than one inch back and forth). As your baby settles, gentle rocking will be enough to keep the calming reflex switched on.

In some traditional cultures, moms bounce their babies all day long. Many wear infants in slings to give them soothing motion with every step. In our culture, tired parents use bouncy seats and exercise balls, car rides, swings, and slings to help their babies find some peace.

Mark and Emma came to my office with their two kids. While I was examining four-year-old Rose, their two-month-old, Mary, startled out of a deep sleep and immediately began to wail. Without missing a beat, Mark scooped her up and began swinging her from side to side, as if he were a metronome. Within twenty seconds, Mary's eyes glazed, her body melted into his chest, and we were able to finish the visit as if she had never made a peep.

5th *S*: Sucking—The Icing on the Cake

Sucking is the glorious fifth *S*. Some babies calm at light speed when put to the breast or given a pacifier. But, for most infants, sucking is the icing on the cake of calming; after a baby has been quieted from the other *S*'s, it brings him into profound tranquility.

It's hard to scream with a pacifier in your mouth, but that's not why sucking is so soothing. Pacifier sucking (*nonnutritive* sucking) triggers the calming reflex. Breast- or bottle-feeding (*nutritive* sucking) also triggers the calming reflex, plus they relieve hunger and release soothing cerebral endorphins, which leads to a rich, sleepy relaxation.

Note: Silicone soothers are helpful, but the all-time, number-one "paci" is a mom's nipple. Moms in some cultures offer the breast up to one hundred times a day!

Your baby won't just enjoy the 5 *S*'s; they will transport her into serenity. But only if you do the *S*'s correctly. Swaddle too loosely, and your baby will struggle harder. Shush too softly, and her yelps will continue. Once she's calm, though, continuing a low level of the *S*'s—quieter sound and slower swinging—will keep the reflex turned on.

The first two *S*'s—swaddling and side/stomach—get the calming process started by restricting flailing as you begin to activate the calming reflex. The third and fourth *S*'s—shushing and swinging—break the crying cycle by fully triggering the calming reflex. Finally, the fifth *S*—sucking—keeps the reflex turned on, guiding your baby to even deeper levels of relaxation.

Like any new skill, the 5 *S*'s ability get better with practice. Many families divide the parenting tasks with moms in charge of feeding and dads becoming the swaddle kings and calming experts.

In Boulder, Colorado, public health nurses gave the *Happiest Baby* DVD, our special white noise CD, and a swaddling blanket to forty-two families with fussy babies. Within days, forty-one of the infants (even two withdrawing from drugs!) were much easier to calm. The one baby who did not improve turned out to have an ear infection. And he calmed with the *S's* once that was treated. Clearly, womb rhythms aren't a cure-all. If your child is hungry or her ear hurts, the *S's* will give only momentary relief.

Some skeptics hear about the 5 *S's* and think, "So what's new? Those techniques are as old as the hills." True, these methods *have* been known for centuries. But what was *never* known before was the existence of the calming reflex.

Note: Not only do parents get better with practice, so do babies! After a week of swaddling, many babies stop their struggles, straighten their arms, and actually begin to calm the instant they're placed on a blanket. It's as if they're saying, "Hey, I remember this! I really like it!"

The *5 S's* Save Lives

The 5 *S's* are now taught by public health programs across the United States and in dozens of other nations. Doctors have adopted this approach for two key reasons: 1) It helps parents feel confident and bond to their babies, and 2) Reducing infant crying and parent exhaustion can save lives and lower health care costs.

Many scientific studies have confirmed that infant crying and parent exhaustion are key triggers for:

• Child abuse: Causing at least 1,500 hospitalizations per year, including 1,200 cases of brain damage and 400 deaths.

• Postpartum depression: Plaguing 10 to 50 percent of new moms and many new dads. Anxiety and depression can lead to breast-feeding failure, accidents, child neglect, the long-term need for medication, and even suicide.

- Unsafe sleep practices: Causing over 3,000 SIDS and suffocation deaths every year.
- Breast-feeding failure: Leading to SIDS, declining infant health, and increased risk of breast and ovarian cancers for mothers.
- Other health problems: Including maternal smoking, car accidents, overtreatment for acid reflux . . . even maternal obesity.

THREE REASONS YOUR BABY MAY HAVE A DELAYED RESPONSE TO THE 5 S'S

Augie was dozing angelically when I arrived at his hospital room to examine him. But the moment I unwrapped him and the cool air hit his skin, he began to howl. I quieted him with tiny jiggles and strong shushing, but as soon as I stopped, he began wailing all over again. I then wrapped him snugly, rolled his struggling body to the side, rocked him, and made a harsh *shhhh* sound . . . right by his ear. Within seconds, Augie was again at ease.

Ten seconds later, however, his cry surfaced one last time.

Was he in pain? Did he need to burp? No, like an exhausted boxer trying to get up off the mat, he just hadn't fully given up his initial protest. After a little more shushing and rocking, Augie finally gave in, and his little body relaxed.

The first few times you use the 5 S's your baby may ignore you or even cry louder . . . even if you do the techniques perfectly! It may take a little time for your child to fully respond to the S's because:

1. *Baby brains have difficulty shifting gears.*
   Your child's immature brain may be so overloaded by

crying and flailing that he has trouble escaping his own frenzy . . . and can't pay attention to you. (Babies usually relent to the 5 S's after a couple more minutes.)

2. *Baby brains are* s-l-o-w.

Around four months, your baby's eyes will quickly follow you as you walk around the room. But in the early months, it may take a few seconds for messages ("I just saw mom move!") to travel from his brain's vision center to its muscle control center ("Okay, eyes, follow her!").

3. *Baby brains get into cycles of crying.*

When your newborn calms with the 5 S's, he may burst into crying again after ten or twenty seconds. That's because the distress is still *cycling* through his nervous system, like strong aftershocks after his little "volcanic eruption." Don't be surprised if it takes a minute—or more—for the upset to finish cycling through and for the calming reflex to guide your baby into sleep.

Once you've mastered these skills, coping with crying may even become *fun!* Soothing *hunger* cries is a joy when you get good at feeding your baby. And using the 5 S's to quickly calm all other wails is just as satisfying.

Note: You might find it helpful to watch *The Happiest Baby* DVD to see the 5 S's in action . . . with real parents and babies.

Finding a *Happiest Baby* Class Near You

Thousands of *Happiest Baby* educators teach baby-calming and sleep-promotion skills to pregnant couples and new parents across the country and around the world—from city dwellers and suburbanites to military dads, foster moms, and parents of preemies and adopted babies.

Surveys of pregnant couples have found that, before taking a *Happiest Baby* class, 40 percent were "somewhat to very worried" about being able to calm their baby's screaming. After the class, the number of worried parents dropped to just 1 percent.

These classes are available in hospitals and clinics across the country. Businesses even offer *5 S's* classes to boost employee loyalty, reduce absenteeism, prevent on-the-job accidents, and lower insurance costs.

If you'd like to find a teacher and class near you, please visit www.happiestbaby.com.

8

$\sim\sim\sim$

1st *S*: Swaddling—
A Feeling of Pure "WRAPture"

MAIN POINTS

- Swaddling is the cornerstone of calming.
- Your fussy baby may resist wrapping, but without it the next *S's* don't work as well.
- Six swaddling myths and misconceptions.
- The perfect swaddle: The *DUDU wrap*.
- Fixing the four common swaddling mistakes.

One evening, Betsy called in tears:

"Around six weeks, my baby, Alex, began having terrible gas pains. At night, she'd scream almost hourly. I tried everything—even a chicken and water diet—but nothing helped."

Betsy asked for some antigas medicine. I suggested she try the 5 *S's* before resorting to medicine, but she was skeptical.

"I didn't use the *S's* the first night. I was afraid swaddling would make Alex uncomfortable. And I still thought she had pain. But I gave in after a really bad night.

"As soon as I began to swaddle Alex and use the doctor's white noise CD, she began getting better. The second night, even before I had finished wrapping, she fell asleep—and slept for seven hours! What really confused me was I could hear her stomach rumbling and knew that she was still having gas, but clearly it was no longer bothering her."

SWADDLING: THE CORNERSTONE OF CALMING

Many parents say that the first time they tried swaddling was a disaster. The baby struggled; they sweated; the hospital nurse frowned. Swaddling a frantic baby feels pretty wrong . . . like you are forcing

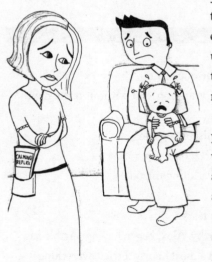

your poor baby to do something she hates. But I strongly encourage you not to give up. Snug wrapping is the key to peaceful days and restful nights.

Note: The first ten times you practice swaddling, do it when your baby is calm or asleep, not when she is fussy and thrashing.

Why does wrapping work so well? Here are three ways it reduces fussing:

1. *The sweet touch of swaddling*

Skin is the largest organ of the body, and touch is our most ancient, calming sense.

We all know how delicious the touch of our baby's skin

feels, but for babies, touch is more than a nice sensation—*it's as lifesaving as milk!* In fact, babies who are given milk but never held or touched may wither and die.

Swaddling is a similar experience to being carried in a sling or cuddled skin to skin, but its big advantage is that it envelops her body with a soft caress that can soothe her for hours when she can't be in your arms.

2. *Swaddling prevents spiraling out of control.*

Wrapping keeps your baby from accidentally whacking herself and getting even more upset. Before birth, your uterus kept her arms from spinning like a windmill. Without those soft walls stopping her flailing, small upsets can quickly escalate. (Have you noticed how much calmer your little one is when she is "wrapped" in your arms?)

3. *Swaddling helps babies pay attention to soothing.*

Crying makes babies feel like their heads are filled with loud warning sounds. Each jerk and startle sets off another alarm. All those rapid-fire jolts cause such chaos that your infant may not even notice your attempts at comforting.

Swaddling reduces those distractions and offers a reassuring embrace that says "It's okay. Mama is taking over now."

The Great Surprise About Swaddling

A big misconception about wrapping is that it quiets fussing. Swaddling prepares your baby for soothing, but wrapping alone rarely turns on the calming reflex. In fact, many babies scream *more* when first bundled!

This struggling may make you think "My baby hates swaddling. I would want my hands free and so does she!" But it's a mistake to think your baby wants the same things you do. You might hate to be swaddled, but you would also hate to live in a womb for nine months or drink milk for every meal. You get my point?

If infants cried because they wanted to free their swaddled hands, calming them would be a snap: Just never wrap them. Unfortunately, as you've probably noticed, the instant your fussy baby is released from swaddling her arms *boing* back up—causing even more screaming!

Please don't lose confidence when your infant fights the wrap. Her resistance means "I'm out of control!" not "I hate this!"

Note: Many parents observe that, after a couple of weeks, their infants learn how nice swaddling feels. They begin to straighten their arms as soon as they're laid on the blanket . . . even before the wrapping begins!

ONCE UPON A TIME: HOW PARENTS USED SWADDLING IN OTHER AGES AND CULTURES

> *I banish from you all tears, birthmarks, flaws, and the troubles of bed-wetting. Love your paternal and maternal uncles. Do not betray your origins. Be intelligent, learned, and discreet. Respect yourself, be brave.*
>
> Ritual instructions spoken when swaddling a baby by the Berber people of Algeria, Béatrice Fontanel and Claire D'Harcourt, *Babies Celebrated*

For thousands of years, moms have swaddled babies. Our ancestors wrapped them in blankets . . . and even secured the bundles with strings and belts. Swaddling is one of the most universal parenting techniques in history. That's because:

• It's safer: Wrapped babies are less likely to wiggle out of their moms' arms and fall.

- It's easy: While a mom works, her baby can be strapped onto her back or slung on a hip.
- It's calming: Babies cry less, which helps everyone around them be happier.

Great Swaddling Moments in History

- Historical records tell us that Alexander the Great, Julius Caesar, and Jesus were all swaddled as babies. (George Washington probably was, too!)
- In Tibet, babies have always been swaddled tightly in blankets. Traditionally, the wrapping is snugged with rope and the baby is secured to the side of a yak to be safely carried as the family treks along rugged mountain paths.
- On the high, windy plains of Algeria, babies have always been swaddled to protect them from evil spirits and disease-provoking drafts.
- During the Middle Ages, European parents kept their babies immobilized in tight, bulky swaddles for the first four to nine months.
- Many Native American tribes carried their babies—papooses—tightly packaged and slung onto their backs. (The 2000 U.S. one-dollar coin displays Sacajawea, Lewis and Clark's Native American guide, with her tiny baby snugly bundled on her shoulders.)

WRAPPING GETS UNRAVELED: WHY MOMS STOPPED SWADDLING . . . CENTURIES AGO

During the Middle Ages, Europeans wrapped their babies for some very good—and some very crazy—reasons. Swaddling was loved because it kept babies warm and quiet. But parents also believed that unwrapped babies might pluck out their own eyes, dislocate their arms, or wind up with bow legs.

Then, in the 1700s, the Enlightenment began and popularized two new trends in Western society: science and democracy. As important as those movements are, they led to two mistaken ideas that led to the abandonment of swaddling for the next three centuries:

MISTAKE 1. Swaddling is useless: In the 1700s, scientists recognized that unwrapped infants never plucked out their eyeballs, dislocated their arms, or had exaggerated leg bowing. From these observations, they wrongly assumed that swaddling was a silly and unnecessary tradition.

MISTAKE 2. Babies need freedom: Our founding fathers (and mothers) wanted all children to live in freedom. Since no animal put their babies in this type of unnatural "bondage," they rejected swaddling as a form of baby "prison."

Within one hundred years, Western parents had all but abandoned snug wrapping. But, as parents unbound their babies, the number that shrieked skyrocketed.

Soon these screams provoked a third mistake. In response to this rising tide of colic, early scientists concluded that these babies were in pain and prescribed the two best pain medicines of the 1800s—gin and opium. It sounds incredible to us today, but fussy babies everywhere were dosed with these powerful anesthetics . . . until the 1970s! And over the past forty years, those strong drugs were replaced by a parade of sedatives, such as phenobarbital and Valium; antispasmodics, such as belladonna; and acid reflux drugs.

SIX SWADDLING MYTH-CONCEPTIONS

Swaddling is as old as the hills, yet there are some common myths and misconceptions that you might read on the Internet about this ancient practice.

1. MEDICAL AUTHORITIES DISCOURAGE SWADDLING.

No! The American Academy of Pediatrics (AAP) recommends swaddling in its books, on its website, and in its child abuse prevention program. In fact, the AAP's last report on reducing sudden infant death syndrome (SIDS) noted "Swaddling, when done correctly, can be an effective technique to help calm infants and promote sleep."

Safe swaddling is also encouraged by the Australian SIDS prevention program, SIDS and Kids; the Canadian Pediatric Society; and the International Hip Dysplasia Institute.

Today, swaddling is taught in hospitals, universities, state and local public health programs and in dozens of other countries.

Note: Swaddling must always be done correctly to avoid overheating, stomach sleeping, loose blankets, and tightness around the hips.

2. SWADDLING RAISES THE RISK OF SIDS.

No! In fact, the top Australian SIDS prevention program recommends swaddling . . . for up to six months!

An Australian study found that swaddled babies sleeping on the stomach had a higher risk of SIDS, but only if they also had a pillow in the crib. A British study reported more SIDS among swaddled babies, but they too found that many SIDS victims were sleeping on a pillow and almost 30 percent were in poor recent health.

3. SWADDLING SHOULD BE STOPPED AT TWO MONTHS.

Two months is actually *the worst* age to stop swaddling! Some doctors worry that a wrapped baby who rolls to the stomach might have trouble lifting his head and breathing. But since proper swaddling reduces a baby's wiggling and rolling, it should actually prevent crib death caused by rolling to the stomach! (You can read more about the prevention of SIDS on page 129.)

Two to four months is the time babies need swaddling the most. It is the peak age of the many dangers triggered by crying and parental exhaustion, including child abuse, postpartum depression, breast-feeding failure, maternal cigarette smoking, car accidents, and infant sleep deaths.

Note: Of course, no baby—wrapped or unwrapped—should ever sleep on the stomach. If your infant can roll while swaddled, consider these three precautions:

WRAP CORRECTLY. Swaddling that is too loose encourages baby rolling.

USE WHITE NOISE. When the room is silent, babies are more apt to wiggle and roll.

PREVENT ROLLING. Ask your doctor about using a smart sleeper or securing your swaddled baby in a *fully reclined* swing during sleep periods.

Does Swaddling *Prevent* SIDS? Probably!

Millions of babies are wrapped, so if it caused SIDS one would expect hundreds of swaddle-related sleep deaths each year. But a study from 2004 to 2012 found fewer than two sleep deaths per year among swaddled babies. And most victims were stomach sleeping or had unsafe, bulky bedding. The authors noted that "reports of sudden unexpected death in swaddled infants are rare."

This extremely low SIDS rate shows that wrapping may actually *prevent* SIDS and suffocation. Australian doctors also found that swaddled babies (sleeping on the back) were one-third less likely to die from SIDS, and a New Zealand study found a similar benefit.

Another recent eight-year study reported on deaths related to sofa sleeping. Babies were brought to the sofa because of crying or for a feeding . . . and then the mom fell asleep. Most of these 1,024 fatalaties were in babies under three months old. I believe that many of these parents would not have fallen asleep in that dangerous location had they used swaddling to keep their babies sleeping longer.

Here are four final strands of evidence that point to wrapping as a way to prevent SIDS and suffocation:

1. Stops rolling: Swaddling makes it hard for babies to flip over. That's important because SIDS risk jumps eight to forty-five times for babies who routinely back sleep, but accidentally roll!

2. Reduces unsafe sleeping: By reducing crying, swaddling lessens a mom's temptation to put her baby to sleep on the stomach. It also may reduce her temptation to bring the baby into her bed.

3. Reduces cigarette smoking: Infant crying can push a mom to restart smoking, which raises the SIDS risk.

4. Boosts breast-feeding: Nursing reduces SIDS risk by up to 50 percent. Swaddling boosts nursing by reducing the crying and exhaustion that leads some women to abandon nursing (because of depression or doubts about the adequacy of their milk).

---

4. SWADDLING INTERFERES WITH BREAST-FEEDING.

No! Swaddling can actually *increase* breast-feeding success.

Swaddling makes it easier to latch your baby on the breast. (That's hard to do when she's crying!) It may also reduce mastitis (by improving sleep and feeding efficacy) and lessen the need for severe dietary changes (often recommended because of infant fussiness). For these reasons, *Happiest Baby* is taught in hundreds of breast-feeding clinics to boost success of poor and at-risk new moms.

The U.S. Centers for Disease Control studied thirty thousand breast-feeding moms to see why women give up nursing early. Women who stopped during the first month usually did so because of technique issues, like nipple pain. Women who gave up nursing after the first month usually said the baby disliked their milk, or they worried they weren't making enough of it. Perhaps, if these moms had better baby-calming skills, they might have continued nursing as long as they had originally planned.

Despite the obvious benefits of the 5 S's, some breast-feeding activists worry that swaddling and the other S's may interfere with nursing. They speculate that this approach a) puts babies into a state of panic, b) leads moms to ignore their babies, instead of holding them skin to skin, and c) reduces nighttime early hunger cues, causing underfeeding.

Fortunately, all these concerns are easily dismissed.

Swaddling doesn't *panic* babies. In fact, it allows upset babies to become calm and alert. Studies also show that wrapping slightly lowers a baby's heart rate. Panic would speed it.

Infant carrying and skin-to-skin contact are wonderful experiences, except during a) sleep, when they become unsafe, and b) inconsolable crying, when they have failed to calm the baby. That's when swaddling comes to the rescue.

Finally, during the early weeks, babies need eight to twelve feedings per day. But that doesn't mean they must eat every two hours all through the night. Your job is to meet your baby's needs *and* to preserve your mental and physical health. As long as you feed lots during the day (when you're wide awake), it's fine to let your newborn have a four-hour stretch of sleep—once or twice a night. It will keep you healthier and happier and improve your nursing success.

5. SWADDLING CAN DANGEROUSLY OVERHEAT YOUR BABY.

No! You never want your baby to be too hot, and, fortunately, several studies show that there is no risk of overheating from swaddling, unless your baby is:

- Bundled in too many layers
- In a hot room
- Wearing a hat

Of course, you should not overdress your baby or overheat the room . . . whether she's swaddled or not. Your best bet it to keep the room at 68°F to 72°F (20°C to 22.2°C). Hats are problematic because they can slip over the face.

In addition to overheating, *overcooling* can raise the SIDS risk. A New Zealand study found unswaddled babies—in cold rooms—had almost four times more crib death.

Warning: Don't Let Your Baby Become a Red-Hot Chili Pepper

Hillary thought her new baby, Rob, needed the room temperature to be the same tropical 98.6°F he loved inside her. But she was taking the fourth trimester idea a bit too far!

Overheating can make babies restless, cause heat rash, and raise the risk of SIDS.

To avoid turning your baby into a hot potato:

- Check the ears and neck. If the ears are red and hot and the neck is sweaty, your baby is too warm. Dress her more lightly or cool the room. If her ears are cold, use a little more clothing or warm up the room.

- Don't overbundle with thick blankets, extra layers of clothing, or hats.
- Never use electric blankets or heating pads. These overheat babies and expose them to electromagnetic radiation.
- In hot weather, use just a diaper and light muslin swaddle. Sprinkle on a dusting of cornstarch powder—never talcum powder—to absorb sweat and prevent rashes.

---

6. SWADDLING CAN CAUSE HIP PROBLEMS.

Not when done correctly! Some doctors warn that wrapping might hurt a baby's hips. Indeed, cultures using *ancient* methods of swaddling (with rigid, fully straightened legs, tightly bound with blankets or ropes) have more infant hip dysplasia and adult hip arthritis.

Fortunately, there have been no reports of increased hip problems over the past decade despite millions of infants having been swaddled. America's top pediatric hip experts, the AAP, the Pediatric Orthopaedic Society of North America, and the International Hip Dysplasia Institute all encourage parents to swaddle . . . *but only when it's done correctly.*

The key is to not swaddle the legs tightly together, like a cigar. "Hip-healthy" wrapping holds the arms very snug, but lets the knees bend and the hips easily flex and open. Safe swaddling is described beginning on page 114.

Note: If your baby has a known hip risk factor, such as breech delivery, club foot, torticollis, a hip *click* noted during a physical examination, or a family history of hip dysplasia, ask the doctor if you should use a triple diaper to keep your baby's hips open for extra protection.

Are Sleep Sacks Safer Than Swaddling? Not Necessarily

Some nurses think sleep sacks are safer than swaddle blankets. They worry that a flat blanket might get loose and cover the baby's face.

Fortunately, a German study found no increased SIDS risk with thin blankets, although SIDS did double with thick blankets and comforters. Dutch researchers also found infant head covering was a risk only for babies sleeping with duvets (17/19 SIDS victims with covered heads were under heavy blankets). For these reasons, the American Academy of Pediatrics allows the use of thin wraps.

What about sleep sacks? One British study showed a smaller SIDS risk using sleep sacks, but I still have concerns. Having the arms free allows your baby to flail, which leads to more crying and less sleep. And they don't stop babies from swinging their arms and rolling into trouble. Sleep sacks with little swaddle wings (to keep the arms restricted) do have risks. A 2014 study reported eight deaths among babies using these sacks.

Bottom line: Sleep sacks are a convenience for parents who have trouble getting the hang of traditional swaddling, but they are probably no safer. And since one has to buy bigger sizes as the infant grows, sleep sacks end up being two to six times more expensive.

Can Swaddling Prevent Postpartum Depression?

Swaddle skeptics often ignore one of its key benefits: reducing serious crying- and exhaustion-related problems, such as postpartum depression (PPD). PPD affects 10 to 50 percent of all new mothers, and up to 25 percent of their partners.

Doctors at Brown University reported that 45 percent of moms with colicky babies develop moderate to severe PPD.

(That's ten times more serious PPD than women whose babies are not screamers!) Supporting that finding, a Boston pediatrician discovered that just twenty minutes of inconsolable crying each day quadruples a woman's risk of developing postpartum depressive symptoms.

Thankfully, swaddling—especialy when used with white noise—reduces crying, boosts sleep and may prevent depression. For this reason, swaddling, and all of the *S's*, are used in PPD prevention and treatment programs.

Note: Swaddling may also reduce other problems triggered by crying and exhaustion, such as child abuse, excessive doctor or emergency room visits, unnecessary acid reflux medicine, fatigue-related car accidents, and mom and baby obesity.

SWADDLING MAKES A COMEBACK!

Twenty years ago, I visited a hospital in northern Italy. I mentioned the missing fourth trimester to the head neonatologist and shared my belief that a worldwide renaissance of wrapping had begun. The director listened patiently, but after I finished, he patted me on the shoulder and said, "I appreciate your passion, but in Italy we believe babies need their hands free to encourage development. We haven't wrapped babies in generations."

Just at that moment, his secretary summoned him for a phone call. No sooner had he left than the head nurse approached me and whispered, "*Il direttore* likes the babies unwrapped, but at the end of the day when he leaves, we bundle them up again!"

For three centuries, Western parents turned their backs on swaddling. But since the release of *The Happiest Baby* there has been a *swaddling explosion*! From a rarity, swaddling has now become the norm . . . because it works.

Why Is Swaddling Banned in Some Day Care Centers?

The state has gone *mad!* We've used swaddling and sound for the past three years and found an amazing difference in the quality of sleep and learning for our infants (and in the sanity and satisfaction of our teachers).

Recently Texas banned blankets of any kind unless we have a permission slip from the infant's pediatrician! But blankets don't kill babies. . . . Poor supervision and training kill babies!

Teacher at Abilene, Texas, Early Head Start

Now that you know how helpful swaddling is, it may surprise you to learn that three states have barred it from day care settings: Minnesota, Pennsylvania, and Texas!

In 2011, a tragically misguided report released by the National Resource Center (a group that develops child care rules for the entire United States) said improper swaddling might cause overheating, suffocation, and hip problems.

I called the NRC to discuss their position and they said childcare workers might not swaddle correctly. (Apparently, the NRC thought these workers were smart enough to learn how to resuscitate a baby who had stopped breathing, but not how to properly swaddle.)

When I asked about the bans, the NRC said they never recommended a ban on wrapping. They had merely advised that swaddling was "not necessary or recommended." They said the states had misinterpreted their comments., but they refused to contact the states to reverse the prohibition.

I am concerned that this flawed policy will lead to more crying, and more death, as:

1. Exhausted caregivers put fussy babies to sleep in unsafe positions.
2. Stressed-out parents abuse their babies.

3. Desolate mothers lapse into depression.

4. Unswaddled babies in day care roll to their stomachs, increasing the risk of SIDS.

THE *DUDU WRAP:* LEARNING TO SWADDLE— STEP BY STEP

The first step to calming any fussy baby is to give her a cozy embrace. That's exactly what swaddling does. Except swaddling has the extra benefit of letting you put your baby down so you can sneak some bonus minutes to relax, cook a meal, or go to the bathroom.

I know it is hard to believe, but when this book came out in 2002, swaddling blankets were almost nonexistent. (Moms in my practice used to sew them themselves!) Now swaddlers are available everywhere . . . in dozens of varieties.

Yet, even though millions of blankets are sold each year, many parents never learn to wrap correctly. That worries me, because incorrect swaddling may accidentally worsen crying or pose a health hazard. Fortunately, safe swaddling is not rocket science. It may be tricky at first, especially if your baby is upset and struggling. (Gulp!) But, after five or ten tries, it will become as easy as changing a diaper.

There are lots of ways to swaddle, but I think the best is a method I learned years ago from a wonderful midwife. It's a four-step approach I call the *DUDU wrap* (Down-Up-Down-Up).

Note: When you're just starting this method it's easier to practice it when your baby is calm or already asleep.

To get ready:

1. Place a light cotton blanket on your bed (use a 44-inch by 44-inch square) and orient it like a diamond, with a point at the top.

2. Fold the top corner down. The top point should end up near the center of the blanket.

3. Place your baby on the blanket, her neck right above the edge of the top fold.

4. Hold her right arm straight at her side. (If she resists, just be patient. The arm will straighten after a moment or two of gentle pressure.)

Now you can start:
1. DOWN
Holding the *right* arm against her side, grab the blanket about four inches from her *right* shoulder. Then, pull it snugly down and across her body. Tuck it under her *left* buttock. (It will look like half of a V-neck sweater.) Next, grab the free blanket, beside her *left* shoulder. Tug it firmly—away from her body—to remove any slack.

Her right arm should now be straight and snug against her side.

(Just as swaddling is the key to calming, this first DOWN is the key to swaddling. Do it snugly . . . or the whole wrap will unravel.)

Note: Don't be surprised if your baby's cries escalate when you start to swaddle! You're not hurting her. She just doesn't realize yet that she's only seconds away from happiness.

2. UP

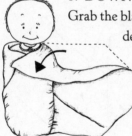

Now, holding her *left* arm against her side, bring the point at the bottom of the blanket straight up and place it on her *left* shoulder. Tuck the blanket edge snugly around the left arm. Again, grab the blanket next to her shoulder and pull it straight out—away from her body—to remove any slack.

Note: The blanket should be loose around her legs, but her arms should be very snug and straight. Bent arms let babies wiggle out . . . and that makes them cry even more.

3. DOWN

Grab the blanket just a few inches from the left shoulder and pull it down—*just a smidge.* The small flap should come down to her upper chest to form the other half of the V-neck. Lightly press that smidge against her breastbone, like you're holding down a ribbon while making a bow.

Note: *Don't* bring this fold all the way down to your baby's feet! It's just brought down to the chest.

4. UP

Holding the smidge on the chest, grab the last free blanket corner and pull it *straight out* (away from her body) to remove any slack. Then, in one smooth motion, lift that corner up *and straight across her forearms . . . like a belt.* The blanket should be big enough so that this part goes all the way around the body. Then, snug it and tuck it into the front of the "belt."

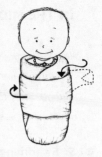

Note: This last step is not straight up . . . it is really up *and across*. The arms will be held snug and straight, but the legs should be loose enough to bend at the knee and open at the hips.

If you're confused at all, watch the three swaddling demonstrations on *The Happiest Baby* DVD or take a lesson from a *Happiest Baby* educator (www.happiestbaby.com). And if you're still struggling, there are many Velcro or zippered pre-made swaddles on the market.

Here's a summary for when you want to do a quick review:

Note: Calming your baby is like dancing with her . . . but she is leading. Start the 5 S's with a little vigor, to mirror her level of upset. Then, lessen the intensity as she begins to settle.

1st *S*: Swaddling

Don't worry if your baby's first reaction is to struggle against the wrapping. Swaddling may not instantly calm her fussies, but it will restrain her flailing so she can pay attention to the next *S's,* which *will* turn on her calming reflex and guide her into serenity.

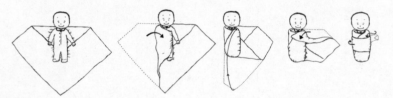

2nd *S*: Side/Stomach

The back is the only safe position for sleep. But the fussier your baby gets, the less happy she'll be on her back. Rolling her to the side or stomach may quickly soothe her. For many babies, this simple step does the trick . . . in under a minute.

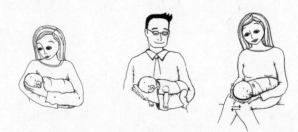

BABY'S CRYING WITH THE *5 S'S*

3rd *S*: Shushing

Shushing may magically make your crying baby feel
at peace. But unless you do it about as loud as her
howls . . . she may not even notice. A womb sound
download or CD with rough, rumbling white noise is a
big help for keeping your baby calm and for boosting
sleep throughout the night.

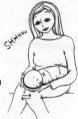

4th *S*: Swinging

Bouncy jiggling can quickly rescue your baby
from a meltdown. Supporting the head and
neck in your open hands, jiggle her head back
and forth in fast, tiny movements (just about
one inch). Once entranced, you can move her—
swaddled—into a smart sleeper or an infant
swing for continual, hypnotic motion. (Before
using a swing, always get your doctor's permission. Make sure
the strap is between your baby's legs, and that the swing is *fully
reclined.*)

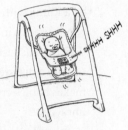

5th *S*: Sucking

Sucking works best after you've already soothed your little one
with the other *S's*. Offering your breast, finger, or a pacifier is like
the icing on the cake of soothing. You can teach
your baby to keep the pacifier in her mouth by
using *reverse psychology:* When she's sucking on
the pacifier, gently tug on it as if you're going to
take it out. (Read more about this in chapter 12.)

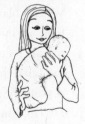

IRON OUT THE WRINKLES: FIXING COMMON SWADDLING MISTAKES

Swaddling is simple, but you'll want to avoid common mistakes:

- Loose wrapping
  A Harvard study found that babies *actually cry more* if they are wrapped loosely!

  The secret of swaddling is keeping the arms snug, while leaving the blanket loose around the knees and hips so they can bend and open easily.
- Swaddling with bent arms
  Some experts insist that infants have their hands up high so they can suck their fingers. But wrapping with bent arms is usually a disaster! It allows the hands to wiggle out, which makes babies cry more . . . and allows the whole wrap to unravel.

  It's true that, during the last month or two of pregnancy, a baby's arms are always bent. However, within two weeks of birth, the arms naturally relax, becoming straighter during calm times and sleep. (Although they do snap back into the bent position during crying.)

  Note: Preemies can be wrapped with bent arms, until they near their due date.
- Letting the blanket touch the cheek
  When a blanket touches the cheek of your hungry baby, it fools her into thinking it's the breast. That can set off the rooting reflex and cause her to cry with frustration when she can't find the nipple. So keep the blanket off the face, by making the swaddle look like a V-neck sweater. (See the *DUDU wrap* instructions beginning on page 114.)
- Your blanket is too small
  Small blankets tend to pop open and unravel. Use a blanket

that's big enough to wrap all around your baby's body—at least 44 inches square.

The Whys About the *S's*: Questions Parents Ask About Swaddling

What a difference a decade makes! In 2002, many parents and grandparents feared that swaddling would deprive their baby of freedom. But today, millions confidently wrap their infants.

Nevertheless, parents still have lots of questions about swaddling. Here are the ones I get asked the most:

1. *When should I start wrapping my baby?*

   Swaddling starts on day one! It makes babies feel like they're "back home."

   Of course, it's also great to put your baby on your chest—skin to skin. But, when skin-to-skin contact fails to calm her cries—or when you're getting sleepy and need to put her down—swaddling is a great help.

2. *Do all babies need swaddling?*

   Some babies are peaceful without swaddling. But even easy infants stay calmer and sleep longer when swaddled. And the fussier a baby is, the more benefit she'll get from wrapping. Swaddling may also reduce your baby's risk of crib death by preventing flipping and keeping her safely on the back.

3. *Does swaddling boost sleep?*

   Yes! Bundling prevents startling, which can wake your baby from sleep. You can boost her sleep even more by playing rumbly white noise *all night long*. (More about that in chapter 15.)

4. *If my baby has never been swaddled, when is it too late to start?*

   You can start wrapping at any time during her first three

months. But be patient. You may have to practice several times before she gets used to it.

5. *My baby loves swaddling, but when should I wean him?*

Wrapping is most valuable during the fourth trimester. After four or five months, most babies are ready to "graduate." If you're unable to wean the swaddle by then, it usually means you need to use a more rumbly, low-pitched white noise all night long.

6. *How many hours a day should my baby be wrapped?*

All babies need time to stretch, be bathed, and get a massage. So you should plan on swaddling only for sleep and crying periods. As the months go by, you'll gradually reduce the wrapping as waking time increases and fussing wanes.

7. *How can I tell if I'm swaddling too tightly?*

Slide your hand between the blanket and your baby's chest. It should feel about as snug as your elastic waistband— at the end of your pregnancy. In truth, a bigger problem than excessive tightness is wrapping too loosely. That can allow the blanket to unravel and cover your baby's head.

8. *How can I tell if my fussy baby needs swaddling or milk?*

Here are a few ways to assess your baby's level of hunger:

TOUCH HER LIPS OR CHEEK. Does her mouth open like a baby bird waiting for a worm? Babies have a supercharged rooting reflex when they get hungry.

GIVE HER A PACIFIER. Does she happily suck for a few minutes, or quickly get mad because she really wants milk?

OFFER MILK. She will suck and swallow vigorously if she is hungry.

Swaddling helps some babies sleep through mild hunger, but really hungry babies wail whether they're wrapped or not.

Note: During the first two weeks, swaddling makes some babies so sleepy they skip a feeding or two. So unwrap your newborn every couple of hours (during the day) to offer a feeding. If she resists waking, a cool wet cloth on her face and body may help to rouse her.

9. *My baby has started rolling over. Should I stop the swaddling?*

If your swaddled infant can roll, make sure you're a) swaddling correctly, b) using a big enough blanket, and c) playing rumbly white noise. These help put babies into a calmer sleep, so they are less likely to roll.

Some doctors stop swaddling as soon as a baby can roll over (unswaddled). But that worries me because it's easier for unwrapped babies to flip over. However, if your baby can roll over despite being swaddled, ask your doctor for permission to securely buckle your swaddled baby into a *fully reclined* swing or to use a smart sleeper with a secure sleep sack.

Note: Sitting too upright in a swing risks allowing a baby's heads falling forward during sleep, creating a suffocation hazard.

10. *Can swaddling lead to pneumonia?*

No! Several studies have shown that wrapped babies breathe normally—albeit slightly faster—and have normal lung function when swaddled. A Turkish study of 186 babies reported more lung infections among wrapped babies; however, a Mongolian study of more than one thousand swaddled babies found no rise in respiratory infections.

11. *Sometimes my baby wakes up unswaddled, with a loose blanket around him. Is that safe?*

Researchers have shown a suffocation risk from loose *bulky* comforters and duvets, but not loose thin blankets. In a review of SIDS deaths over an eight-year period (during which millions of babies slept swaddled), not a single death was attributed to the unraveling of a *light* swaddling blanket. Nevertheless, you don't want *any* loose blankets around your baby. So make sure to swaddle correctly.

12. *A lactation nurse told me that babies need their hands free at night to give early hunger cues and to self-soothe. Is that right?*

Not really. Swaddling may cover over the earliest hunger cues, but when a baby gets truly hungry she'll definitely wake and call for her meal.

Regarding self-soothing: Fetuses easily suck their fingers because the walls of the womb direct their hands right to the mouth. But, during the first few months, babies lack the coordination to keep their fingers in the mouth. You can let your infant practice her finger-sucking skills—all day long— but at night, it's better to wrap them snugly . . . and offer a pacifier.

Bottom line: Feed your baby lots during the day. But if she's growing well, nursing (and your mental attitude) will be better if you can sleep four hours, twice a night.

13. *Can my baby become dependent on swaddling?*

Swaddling twelve hours a day is not excessive; it's actually a 50 percent cutback from what you gave to her every day in your womb! By four or five months, your baby will be able to smile, push herself up, and roll over, and she'll no longer need wrapping to stay calm. That's when weaning swaddling will be easy.

14. *Does wrapping block a baby's ability to learn about the world?*

Actually, babies pay better attention when their arms aren't in constant motion. Swaddling helps them learn about the world without being distracted by shudders and startles.

15. *Shouldn't children be allowed to be free and not bound up?*

Freedom is wonderful, but with freedom comes responsibility. Once your baby can calm herself, she has earned the right to be unwrapped. But, during the first three or four months, many newborns can't handle the great big world without some cozy swaddling.

A PARENT'S PERSPECTIVE: TESTIMONIALS FROM THE TRENCHES

All newborns stay calmer and sleep longer when they're swaddled. Here are some of their stories:

"Sophia had problems nursing when she was born. Our nurse practitioner advised me to use a special device to supplement her feedings. So I taped this tiny tube to my breast and inserted it into her mouth, along with my nipple.

"After about three weeks, Sophia became increasingly fussy. During feedings, she'd scream and flail, dislodging both my nipple and the tube. Despite my frustration, I stuck with it until right before her two-month checkup. That night she was worse than ever. She thrashed, yanked the tube, and mangled my nipple. I swore I would never feed her that way again.

"At her checkup, I told the doctor about my struggles, and he said four words that changed everything: "Don't forget about swaddling." We had wrapped Sophia initially but stopped after a few weeks because she fought it so much. We thought she hated it, but we had misread her signals.

"That afternoon, I tightly bundled her and tried nursing (without the tube). The most extraordinary thing happened: She breast-fed calmly and intently . . . as though she had never had a problem! After that, feeding Sophia was a breeze. Now, at three months, we swaddle her only for sleep or if she's having a really fussy day."

Beth and Colin, parents of Sophia

"The day after Marie-Claire was born, she was crying. Not one of those sweet little newborn squeals, but a really powerful bellow. I was shocked that a one-day-old could make such a sound!

"Just then the doctor came into our room. He casually walked to the bassinet, picked our baby up, and wrapped her like a burrito. Then, putting her on his lap, he made a loud *shhhh* right by her ear. She calmed almost instantly! We were astonished. But, once we learned how to shush and swaddle her, Marie-Claire became the most content baby on the planet!"

Renée and Al, parents of Marie-Claire, Esmé, and Didier

9

~~~~~~

2nd *S*: Side/Stomach—
Your Baby's Feel-Good Position

MAIN POINTS

• The side/stomach position turns on the calming reflex . . .
and turns off the upsetting Moro reflex.
• Infant carriers: Ancient wisdom makes a comeback.
• The reverse-breast-feeding hold and other great ways to
cuddle your baby.

Dugger watched intently as I held his daughter Bobbie. The moment she cried, I placed her cheek in my palm and rolled her small body to rest her chest and stomach against my forearm. Bobbie calmed almost in mid-scream. Then I jiggled her up and down—like a car going over cobblestones—and she eased into sleep in about two minutes.

Dugger later told me, "Football was my favorite sport when I was a boy, and I carried the ball as if it were a treasure. But I never would have felt okay handling Bobbie like that if I hadn't seen you do it. Now I carry Bobbie like a football every day and I am much better at stopping her tears and helping her fall asleep."

In real estate, the key rule is location, location, location. In baby soothing, it's position, position, position.

You know that the back is the *only* safe position for sleeping, but did you know it's also the worst position for calming crying? Most babies happily lie on the back when they're in a peaceful mood, but they *hate* it when they get cranky. In my experience, about 15 percent of all babies are position-sensitive little bugs and simply rolling them to the side or draping their tummy over your shoulder or forearm quickly switches on their calming reflex.

WHY DO THE SIDE AND STOMACH POSITIONS MAKE BABIES HAPPY?

Before birth, your fetus never laid flat on his back. Lying on the side, curled into the *fetal position*—head down, spine rounded, knees pressed against his belly—activated position sensors in his muscles and inner ear to keep his calming reflex turned on. (Even adults feel more serene when they're coiled into the fetal position.) Babies who wiggle too much in the womb can dangerously kink the umbilical cord with their twisting arms and legs.

Holding your fussy baby on his back is a bit like calming *and pinching* him . . . at the same time! That's because upset babies feel insecure on their backs, as if they're being dropped. That position triggers the Moro, or falling, reflex, which makes crying babies fling their arms out and yelp even more. On the other hand, rolling your baby to the side or stomach causes his position sensors to send out a soothing message: "Don't worry. Everything's *fine!*"

Note: Some infants are so sensitive to position that even rolling them slightly—from the side *toward the back*—panics them. Conversely, rolling them slightly—from the side *toward the stomach*—is calming.

A Position for Life: Helping Babies Avoid SIDS

For unhappy babies, lying on the side or stomach can be as soothing as cookies and milk. However, he should *always* be placed on his back when he is out of your arms.

Begun in 1994, the AAP's Back to Sleep campaign has reduced SIDS deaths by more than half, just by advising parents to only allow their babies to sleep on the back for the early months. (FYI, 80 percent of SIDS occurs during the first four months, and 90 percent by six months.)

ONCE UPON A TIME: HOW PARENTS USED THE SIDE/STOMACH POSITION IN OTHER AGES AND CULTURES

> *Among the Inuit (Alaskan natives), a very deep hood is used as a baby bag and serves as an extension of the womb. The newborn lives in a heated climate, completely buried inside the mother's clothing, and curled up like a half-moon.*
>
> Béatrice Fontanel and Claire D'Harcourt, *Babies Celebrated*

Few parents around the world place their infants on their backs, but when they do, they put them on a curved surface, not a flat one. The arc of a small blanket suspended from a tree or tripod puts a baby back into the familiar and reassuring rounded fetal position, encouraging tranquility and sleep.

In most traditional cultures, babies spend a large part of the day just "hanging out." Their moms, sisters, aunts, and neighbors carry them in baskets and sheets, on various parts of their bodies . . . for up to twenty-four hours a day.

- The Lapp people of Greenland carry babies curled up in cradles draped on one side of a reindeer (counterbalanced on the other side by a heavy sack of flour).
- The !Kung San tribe of the Kalahari Desert carry their infants in leather slings all day long. They keep them in a semi-sitting position, because they believe that posture encourages the baby's development.
- In parts of Indonesia, loving moms never let their babies stretch out completely. In that culture, lying flat is the feared position of the dead. (Even new moms must sleep sitting up for forty days after delivery to evade evil spirits who prey on people weakened by illness or injury.) These new parents compactly bundle their infants in a seated position and suspend them from the ceiling to sleep like little floating Buddhas.
- The Efé tribe of pygmies, living in the Democratic Republic of Congo, hold babies upright or curled in their arms all day long, even while they are sleeping. However, since it's such a big effort to do all this carrying, babies are passed back and forth among friends and relatives about eight times an hour during the early months!

Infant Carriers: Ancient Wisdom Makes a Comeback

People used to think that moms with baby carriers were granola people and hippies . . . but now I think women are weird if they don't use one.

Debra, mother of twins Audrey and Sophia

Slings and baby carriers offer a delicious blend of touch, movement, and sound. And they leave our hands free for other jobs. I suspect that these precious little folds of cloth may be among the first "tools" ever invented.

Despite their practicality, slings were discarded by Western culture centuries ago. During the late 1800s, pushing a stroller (referred to back then as a *baby buggy* or *pram*) was seen as more ladylike than walking with a baby slung over your shoulder.

In 1894, Emmett Holt, the "Dr. Spock" of his day, cautioned mothers not to spoil fussy babies by picking them up and rocking them to sleep.

In the 1970s, babies in slings were still a countercultural oddity. But in the 1980s, new scientific studies—and the revival of other time-honored practices such as breast-feeding, practicing yoga, and eating organic food—encouraged parents to revisit the ancient act of baby wearing.

In 1986, researchers in Montreal found that carrying babies for three hours a day (in a mom's arms or a sling) reduced fussing by 43 percent. (Unfortunately, carrying by itself wasn't sufficient to reduce crying in intense, colicky babies.)

We still love strollers for transporting heavy babies on long outings. But imagine what it's like to be in a stroller from your infant's perspective: stuck in a bucket seat, unable to see, touch, or hear you very well. No wonder babies adore slings; they are enveloped in the rich presence of our warmth, scent, movement, touch, and sound. Today, infant carriers have been saved from the brink of extinction. In fact, they're so much a part of our culture that it now seems odd for a mom or dad *not* to wear their baby!

When you buy a sling, here are a few hazards to avoid:
• Make sure it's not too deep: Your baby should sit high enough for you to see his face. (Babies can suffocate if allowed to sink into the bottom of the bag.)

- Support the back and chin: If your baby's face falls forward, toward his chest, it may be hard for him to breathe or cry for help.
- Prevent falling: Hold your little one snugly enough so that he can't slide out.
- Avoid hot food: Never carry your baby when you're handling hot food or liquids.

THE WINNING SIDE: USING POSITION FOR SOOTHING

Here are a few great ways to treat your baby to the calming pleasure of the side or stomach position:

Reverse-Breast-Feeding Hold

This is my favorite way to carry crying babies while I'm bouncing them into calm. It's easy, comfortable, and perfectly supports their head and neck.

1. With your baby lying on his back (swaddled is best), place your palm on the front of his diaper.
2. Roll him onto your forearm, so his stomach rests against your arm (your upper arm and elbow securely supporting the head and neck) and bring him in to your body, lightly pressing his back against your chest.

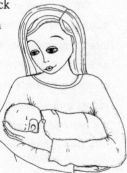

Football Hold

Soothing babies, mid-squawk, with the football hold is one of the greatest baby "magic tricks" of all time. (This is like the reverse-breast-feeding hold, but with the head in your hand.)

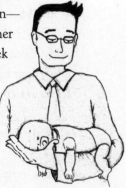

1. With your baby lying on her back (swaddled if fussy), place your hand on her chin— your thumb on one cheek and your other fingers cradled against her other cheek and temple—supporting the head like a chin strap.
2. Gently roll her onto your forearm, snugly cushioning her chest and stomach against your arm. Let her cheek rest in your palm and out-stretched fingers. Her groin will be near your elbow while her legs will dangle, straddled over your arm.

Over-the-Shoulder Hold

Simply lifting your baby to an upright position can often have a strong, soothing effect.

1. Hoist your fussy baby up onto your shoulder.
2. Let the weight of his body press his stomach against your shoulder.

That extra tummy touching makes this hold doubly comforting. (Swaddling your baby before putting him over your shoulder will give you better control and help him stay asleep when you move him off your shoulder to the bassinet.)

Have fun discovering the position that makes your baby the happiest.

The Whys About the S's: Questions Parents Ask About the Side/Stomach Position

1. *Where should I put my baby's hands when he's on his side?*

   Your baby's arms should be placed straight along his body. Even with a snug wrap, there's enough wiggle room to allow your baby to move his lower arms and hands a little bit forward to find his most comfortable position.

2. *Can my baby's arm ever "go to sleep" if he's lying on his side?*

   No. Arms only fall asleep when there's pressure on the "funny bone" (that little notch on the side of the elbow, directly over the ulnar nerve). A swaddled baby never has pressure on that area.

3. *If babies miss the fourth trimester womb sensations, would it make sense to put them upside down?*

   Well, that's an interesting thought, but the answer is no. The womb is filled with fluid so, your fetus actually floats . . . nearly weightlessly. Once born, the buoyancy is gone and being upside down would cause too much pressure, as blood pools in your baby's head.

4. *If I am bed sharing, is it okay for my baby to sleep on the side?*

   When moms bring their babies into their beds, the baby often falls asleep on their side, after a nursing. Unfortunately, that's not a great idea. Studies have shown that side-sleeping babies have a higher risk of SIDS. From the side they can easily roll to the stomach, which raises the risk of SIDS and suffocation.

A PARENT'S PERSPECTIVE: TESTIMONIALS FROM THE TRENCHES

This fussy baby was "beside" himself with joy when his parents put him in his feel-good position:

> Crystal and Rob were confused. At the hospital, Crystal was told to have Max sleep on his back, but when her mom came to visit she gave the opposite advice. "We argued about the best position for my baby's sleeping. He had a really hard time settling when he was flat on his back. I had to pat him for fifteen to twenty minutes until he finally drifted off, and even then he'd still wake every three hours.
>
> "My mom said I should let him sleep on his stomach. I tried it, and he did sleep more soundly in that position, but I was terrified that he might stop breathing.
>
> "When I discussed this with my doctor, he said there was a way I could get the good sleeping of the stomach position with the safety of back sleeping: swaddling! He advised wrapping Max—arms straight and snug—before putting him to sleep on his back. I was thrilled because it helped him sleep as well as my mother's stomach-down position, but was much safer."

10

3rd *S*: Shushing—
Your Baby's Favorite
Soothing Sound

MAIN POINTS

• Story of *shhhh:* The calming sound that babies taught . . . us!
• Four white noise mistakes to avoid.
• Perfect pitch: Picking the best sound for your baby.
• Can noise machines hurt a baby's hearing?

> *My young husband walked our crying baby up and down,*
> *making that shshshshshing sound of comfort that parents*
> *know only too well.*
>
> Eliza Warren, *How I Managed My Children from*
> *Infancy to Marriage*, 1865

As I was making rounds at a local hospital, I saw Sabrina and Yves trying to calm their crying newborn. Both skilled and caring parents, Yves had wrapped the baby snugly and placed her on her side, and

Sabrina was softly whispering in her ear, "It's okay. It's okay." She even offered the baby a pacifier, but nothing helped.

I asked if I could try soothing the baby. Sabrina describes what happened next:

Soleyl had been inconsolable for her first two days of life. After Dr. Karp offered to help, he bent over Soleyl's bassinet, with his face near her ear, and emitted a harsh, continuous "shooshing" sound for about ten seconds. That was it! Soleyl stopped crying almost instantly and remained peaceful for the next two hours.

Of course, one *shhhh* won't keep a baby calm forever, but it was exactly what was needed to capture Soleyl's attention long enough for Sabrina's other calming tricks to work.

WHY DOES *SHHHHING* MAKE BABIES SO HAPPY?

"Tiptoe! The baby is sleeping!" is a warning spoken by millions of new parents all around the world. At first glance, it makes sense—after all, we find quiet rooms restful—but infants are different: *Silence actually drives them crazy!* Hours of quiet can push babies into screaming. It's as if they're begging, "Please, someone make a little noise!"

(Adults also calm with sound. We find deep, rumbly noise, such as rain falling on the roof, trees rustling in the wind, and ocean waves peaceful and relaxing.)

Annette's family joke was that she calmed her baby, Sean, with white nose so often that she should call him "*Shhhh*-ean"!

When I asked Nancy and Gary to guess what their baby, Natalie, heard inside the womb, Nancy said it was probably her shouting, "Hey, Gary, get over here!"

Nancy was partly right. It turns out that rumbly white noise perfectly imitates womb sounds. Fetuses also hear their mom's voice plus other "outside" sounds. But these sounds filter in and out over the daily soundtrack of a loud, continuous symphony of *shhhh*.

How do we know that's what fetuses hear? In the early 1970s, doctors placed tiny microphones into the wombs of women in labor and measured the sound. They noted that wave upon wave of blood surging through the arteries made a thunderous, rumbling noise. The scientists measured this sound at 75 to 92 decibels . . . louder than a vacuum cleaner!

But some parents worry, might that rough roar overwhelm a baby and make her fuss even more? Interestingly, although the womb sound is cranked way up, *your fetus doesn't hear it that loud.* That's because she is packed in water; her ear canals are plugged with waxy vernix; she has fluid in her middle ear; and her eardrums are thick and stiff. All of these factors dampen the intensity of the sound she actually hears.

So imagine your baby's shock when she emerges from the world of loud, quadraphonic uterine whooshing into your quiet world of

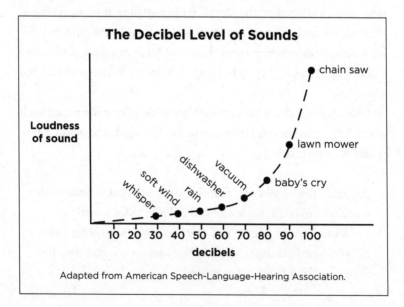

The Decibel Level of Sounds

chain saw

lawn mower

vacuum

dishwasher

baby's cry

soft wind

rain

whisper

Loudness of sound

10 20 30 40 50 60 70 80 90 100

decibels

Adapted from American Speech-Language-Hearing Association.

whispering and empty rooms. Her muffled hearing makes your house seem even more stark.

Note: Within a few weeks, your baby's hearing greatly improves as fluid in the middle ear disappears and her eardrum transforms from the consistency of thick paper to thin cellophane that can vibrate with any distant noise.

ONCE UPON A TIME: HOW PARENTS USED *SHHHHING* IN OTHER AGES AND CULTURES

Did you ever get shushed by a grade school teacher? For millennia, humans have used a hissy *shhhh* (or *ssss* or *pssst*) to tell someone to be quiet. This sound may well be one of the very few "words" understood by people *in every corner of the globe.*

Oddly, the calming effect of shushing may be something that *babies taught us!* In the early mists of human history, cave-moms may have accidentally shushed their wailing babies and been shocked— and pleased—when it instantly soothed the cries.

Once one Stone Age mom learned this trick, she probably couldn't wait to share it with her friends. Over millenia, the discov-

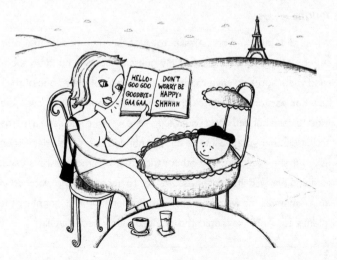

ery and teaching of this fast-acting technique was likely repeated in every tribe and village around the world.

In fact, *shhhh* was so successful in stopping baby crying that it eventually grew from being just a sound to becoming a real part of our vocabulary. Today, many languages incorporate the *shhhh*, *sssss*, or *ch* sound into the word used to say *silence*.

chup (Urdu)	*shuu* (Vietnamese)
chutee (Serbian)	*soos* (Armenian)
tzrch (Eritrean)	*teeshina* (Slovenian)
hush, silence (English)	*toosst* (Swedish)
hushket (Arabic)	*chupraho* (Hindi)
sheket (Hebrew)	*shuh-shuh* (Chinese)
stille (German)	*sessizlik* (Turkish)

Even the Japanese use *shhhh* as the root of their request for quiet: *shizukani* (although as a lover of Japanese food, I might have guessed it would be "shu-shi.")

The Story of *Shhhh:* The Calming Sound That Babies Taught . . . Us

When did moms—from Alaska to Albania—first notice that this strange sound soothed babies? My guess is that one hundred thousand years ago, two cave-moms were eating lunch when one of their new babies started to shriek. In response, her mom leaned over and tried to calm her with loud squawking—the way she had seen a mama crow quiet her young. But the baby continued to cry. Her friend then asked if she could try a soothing trick that her mom always used. Handing her wild little *Infantasaurus rex* to her friend, she watched in amazement as the woman made a strong, harsh *shhhh* . . . right by the infant's ear. And, like magic, the infant suddenly became calm!

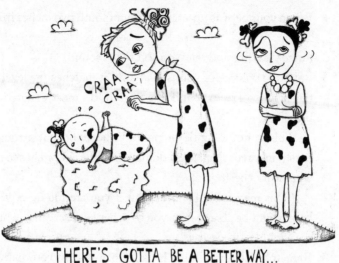

THERE'S GOTTA BE A BETTER WAY...

LEARNING HOW TO *SHHHH* WITH THE BEST OF THEM

As a nurse walked by Paula's hospital room, the door popped open and out came a frazzled dad, pushing a bassinet holding his red-faced, screaming baby. To soothe the little girl, the nurse lovingly leaned her face down near the baby and gave a shush like a burst steam pipe.

I'm confident that, had she continued it a few moments longer, the baby would have calmed. But the baby's father quickly yanked the bassinet away. Glowering at the nurse, he blurted, "How dare you tell my daughter to shut up!"

Of course, she was not telling the baby to shut up. But the dad was understandably incensed because he didn't realize the nurse was talking to the baby in a "different language."

In our language, *Adult-ese*, a loud *"shhhh"* is a rude utterance meaning "shut up." But in *Baby-ese*, *"shhhh"* is a beautiful greeting that all infants recognize and adore!

Here's how to join the worldwide club of parents who shush:

1. When your baby is upset, place your mouth two inches from her ear.
2. Purse your lips and release a soft *shhhh* sound.
3. Raise the volume of your *shhhh* until it matches the level of the crying. (Try to sound like the world's most irritated librarian.)

   This is not a gentle or polite little sound but a rough, harsh, insistent *shhhh*. Try doing it at different pitches to see what works best.

   (This may feel a bit rude, but if you are too quiet your baby won't be able to hear you over her loud screams, which are a jolting *100 decibels!*)
4. Remember, baby calming is like dancing—but your baby is leading. Soften your *shhhh* as the cries lessen and she starts to relax.

Calming your baby with the strong *shhhh* isn't the end of your job; continued moderate white noise will help keep her from sliding back into screaming. (Use white noise for all sleep and crying periods. Remember, your baby was serenaded with sound 24/7 for the past nine months.)

Note: It's fun to teach your older kids how to *shhhh* so they can be more involved in the baby care. They'll feel so proud when they can calm the cries . . . just like Mommy!

Mira and Milu were delighted at how well shushing soothed three-week-old twins Misha and Mihailo: "We'd never have thought the twins would like such an annoying sound, but the louder they cry, the louder they want our shushing to be. We lessen the intensity only after they start to quiet down.

"Shushing makes us pretty dizzy. So when the boys need it for longer periods we play a download of specially engineered sound to substitute for our flagging lung capacity."

FOUR WHITE NOISE MISTAKES YOU WANT TO AVOID

White *light* is made by mixing together all different colors of light. (A rainbow is caused by cracking white light back into all the individual hues). Similarly white *noise* is a mix of all different pitches of sounds blended together.

White noise is a great tool to soothe fussing and boost sleep. But there are some common misunderstandings about how to use it. Some parents think:

1. *My baby sleeps so well, she doesn't need white noise.*

   Even for easy babies, white noise is a must. It makes good sleep even better. And it helps prevent the sleep disasters that may ruin your life between four and twelve months!

   It is very common for an infant's sleep to suddenly *fall apart* after the fourth trimester. That's because: a) the calming reflex fades away, b) babies become super-social and wake up when they hear little noises in the middle of the night, c) they are weaned off being swaddled, and 4) they are teething. All four factors lead to a *surge* in sleep problems . . . just when you thought you had it nailed.

   Using the right white noise will help you sidestep these problems. Within weeks your little one will link the sounds with the pleasure of sleep. *Oh, yeah, I recognize that sound. . . . Now I'll have a nice little snooze.* As she passes through infancy she'll be able to sleep despite *outside* distractions, such as TVs and passing trucks, or *inside* distractions, such as teething pain, mild colds, slight hunger. (Read more on white noise and sleep in chapter 15.)

   Note: *Don't use white noise all day long.* Hearing the normal home sounds, for many hours a day, will help your child master the nuances of all the interesting sounds around her, such as speech, music, and so forth.

2. *All white noise sounds—wave, rain, nature sounds—work equally well.*

People talk about white noise as if it's just one thing. But there are actually two types of white noise—high pitch and low pitch—and they have *totally opposite effects!*

High-pitch white noise is harsh, hissy, whiney, and annoying—think sirens, alarms, beepers, screams. These sounds are great for getting your attention (and calming baby crying), *but they're terrible for sleep.*

On the other hand, low-pitch sound is droning and hypnotic—think the monotonous rumble of a car and planes; rain on the roof; or listening to a boring lecture. That sound is terrible for getting attention, but it's fantastic for lulling us to sleep.

Interestingly, womb sounds start out harsh and hissy, *but* the velvet walls of the womb and the sea of amniotic fluid around your baby filter out the high-pitch frequencies, leaving just a deep, thunderous rumble.

Furthermore, continuous sounds, like hair dryers or rain on the roof, are much more effective than heartbeat, ocean waves, and nature noises.

Note: Parents intuitively use the right pitch to soothe their baby's cries. They start by making a loud, hissy *shhhh* sound and then gradually lower the pitch and volume as their little one relaxes into sleep.

3. *The sound must be played as quietly as possible.*

When your baby cries, you have to: first, *turn on* the calming reflex, and second, keep it turned on.

To turn it on, use a strong hissy sound that's as loud as the crying. Vacuum cleaners rumble at 75 dB and hair dryers roar at 90 dB. But your baby puts them all to shame! Her wails shoot out at 100 dB, or more! That's like a power lawn mower sound blasting just inches from her own ear! No wonder quiet shushing rarely calms screaming; they're so loud they can't even hear us.

Once the outburst starts to settle, keep the calming reflex turned on by playing a rumbly sound, about the intensity of a gentle shower (65 to 70 dB). I particularly recommend using a smart sleeper that automatically boosts the noise during crying bouts and lowers it to a deep, rumbly sound as babies calm.

PERFECT PITCH: PICKING THE RIGHT SOUND FOR YOUR BABY

Making a continuous, loud shush can make you faint from hyperventilation! That's why clever parents have invented other ways to make the sound their babies need.

Some Amazonian Indians use baby slings decorated with monkey bones that rhythmically rattle with every step their mom takes. Parents in our culture may not have access to monkey bones, but we do have dozens of other sound substitutes, including exhaust fans, white noise, noisy swings, buzzing bassinets, and the most dangerous, expensive, and polluting sound machine of all—car rides!

It's worth putting some thought into your sound choice because most white noise machines, apps, and downloads are so hissy they can actually ruin the baby's sleep . . . and *yours*! (Especially if played on tinny phone or computer speakers.)

Here are a few tips to help you create the perfect shush solution:

• Measure the sound intensity. Download a sound meter app on your phone and measure the sound right by your baby's ear. Aim for 80 to 90 dB to calm screams and around 65 dB for sleep.

- White noise is great for soothing screams in the car. And it's perfect on trips to boost your baby's sleep in a hotel or relative's home, despite disturbing new sights, sounds and smells.
- Use sound for all naps, *all* nights, for at least the first year to help your baby sleep longer and better. (Read more about sound and sleep in chapter 15.)

Note: The *Happiest Baby* white noise CD/download contains sounds that are specially engineered. Some are high pitch, perfect for quieting colic. And some filter out the hiss, and amp up the low rumbling sounds, perfect for sleep.

How Rumbly Is the Womb? Try It Yourself

Want to know what your baby heard in the womb? Try this:

Run the water into your bathtub—full blast. Notice how loud it is. Is it high pitched or rumbly? When the tub is almost full, get in, while the water is still running. Now, dunk your head under the water. Does the noise become more thunderous? Under water the sound is similar to the deep rumble your fetus heard in the womb. No wonder babies—and tired adults—sleep better with sound engineered to remove hissing (especially if the sound is played on tinny little speakers).

CAN NOISE MACHINES HURT A BABY'S HEARING?

In 2014, a study of sound machines kicked up a lot of questions about white noise. Researchers tested fourteen machines (marketed

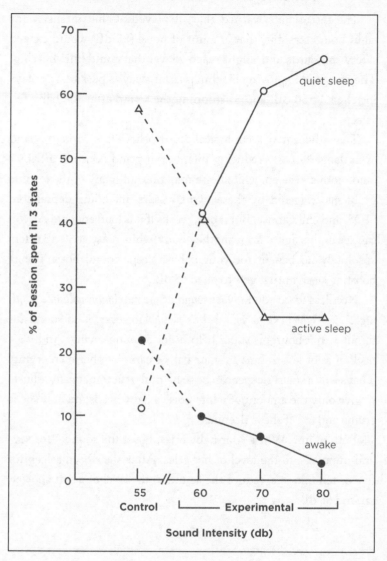

specifically for sleeping babies), placed twelve inches from the babies' heads, and cranked them to max volume. When they measured how much sound reached the baby they found that three devices exceeded 85 dB.

The researchers warned that, if played at that intensity for eight hours straight, that amount of noise (85 dB) would exceed safety standards and might reach a level that could hurt hearing. They advised 1) moving machines as far away as possible, 2) playing them at 50 dB, and 3) stopping the sound after the baby fell asleep.

That advice may seem logical, but I believe it is wrong . . . and even dangerous. By reducing infant crying and boosting a baby's (and mother's) sleep, white noise may prevent many of the terrible problems triggered by these two stressors, including depression, SIDS, and child abuse. But it only works if it is loud enough! As you can see in this figure from another study, white noise at 50 dB offers absolutely no benefit for your baby's sleep. Sound doesn't start boosting sleep until it gets to 60 to 65 dB.

Needless to say, don't *blast sound at the maximum volume . . . all night . . . right next to your baby's head.* However, loud sound for minutes (not hours) is super helpful for calming crying. And it's a heck of a lot *less* trauma to your baby's ears than her own crying! That's why a smart sleeper can be so helpful. It automatically adjusts to give only the amount of white noise a baby needs: more if she is crying and less if she is sleeping.

Bottom line: When your baby cries, boost the sound—for several minutes—to the level of her cries. After she's been asleep for five or ten minutes, reduce the sound to the level of a soft shower, around 65 dB.

Tessa and the Vacuum Cleaner

At five, Tessa was a "pistol"—smart, funny, and intense. But during her first weeks of life, she just couldn't handle her passions, and she would get as wild as a hurricane during her bouts of colic. Her parents, Eve and Todd, wrapped her, walked her, and took her on long car rides, but nothing quelled the crying.

One afternoon, Tessa was wailing but Eve couldn't hold her because she had to get the house ready for company. So she put her crying baby in a little Moses basket and began to vacuum. Amazingly, the instant the vacuum was switched on, Tessa got stone silent!

Eve bolted over and found her sweetly sleeping, her body totally relaxed. Tessa wasn't sleeping *despite* the ruckus; she was sleeping *because* of it!

Eve and Todd began to joke that Tessa was receiving secret messages from the planet Hoover. From then on her parents used the vacuum cleaner whenever their little girl had a meltdown. This calming trick was so predictable that they took great pleasure in inviting friends over during Tessa's fussy time . . . just to watch the show!

Throughout the first year, whenever Eve had to take Tessa to work with her, she brought along a little portable vacuum to settle her in for a good long nap.

The Whys About the S's: Questions Parents Ask About Shhhhing

1. *I was told white noise can overwhelm my baby and push her into neurological* shutdown. *Is that true?*

    Not at all! Rather than stressing babies, white noise soothes them.

    It lowers a baby's heart rate (a sign of *reduced* stress) and is even used to calm infant crying during painful blood tests.

    As mentioned earlier, even strong white noise is less

stressful than the 100 dB sound of the baby's own screaming.

2. *My baby sleeps fine with just swaddling. Does he still need
sound?*

Yes. Even in your wonderful situation, white noise is useful: a) It will help your baby sleep *even better,* and b) it will
prevent sleep problems during the first year triggered by
growth spurts, colds, and teething.

3. *Can white noise hurt a baby's hearing?*

No, as long as you follow certain precautions: Keep it at a
reasonable level and use it only during crying and sleep.
Studies that exposed baby rats to *nonstop* noise—not a second of quiet—for a long time (the equivalent of the first two
years of a human baby's life) found no enduring problems.
(These über-exposed rats had mildly delayed auditory dis-
crimination that resolved after the researchers turned off the
sound.)

Bottom line: White noise is great, but your baby needs
many hours a day *without white noise* to learn the subtleties of
your voice and home sounds.

4. *Can babies get addicted to white noise?*

If by *addicted* you mean that your baby will grow to love
the sound and expect to hear it all night, then *he's already addicted* from the constant sound he enjoyed in the womb. And
even playing it eighteen hours a day is a huge cutback from
what he had in the womb.

But please don't think being "addicted" to this sound is a
problem. After all, most of us are so "addicted" to beds and
pillows, we'd never even consider staying at a hotel that
didn't provide them!

White noise is a great sleep cue because you have total
control over it. It will be easy for you to wean your baby
whenever you want.

5. *Which sound works the best to calm cranky babies: a heart-beat, a lullaby, or* shhhh*?*

One common myth is that babies are calmed by their mom's heartbeat in the womb. Actually, the uterus is so far away from the heart that babies probably never hear it.

Music can lull babies (and adults) into relaxation, but it's not great for calming screams. And, used all night, music's changing tones can actually disturb sleep.

By far, the best sound for calming crying is a continuous, strong white noise that mimics the loud *shhhh* of your womb.

6. *Is it okay to use a white noise app from my phone?*

Yes and no. I have two worries about smartphones: a) they give off microwave radiation, and b) the speakers are tiny and tinny and make high, hissy sounds that can interfere with sleep. Try using a CD or download of deep rumbly sound, played on a good speaker. Or try a smart sleeper that automatically adjusts the sound and intensity of noise to the exact level your baby needs.

Note: If you do use your phone, make sure it's in airplane mode.

7. *When should I wean my baby off white noise?*

Some parents mistakenly assume that they should wean the baby as soon as possible. But it's best to use it for at least the first year to help your little one sleep through teething and growth spurts. (For advice on weaning babies off white noise—and all the 5 S's—see chapter 15.)

8. *If I shush too much, will it lose its effectiveness?*

You might expect babies to get bored with sound, but they don't. Like their long-term love affair with milk, white noise continues to be a favorite comfort for years and years. (Many adults even use white noise to help them sleep.)

A PARENT'S PERSPECTIVE: TESTIMONIALS FROM THE TRENCHES

Discovering different *shhhhing* sounds is an inspired example of parental ingenuity! Some moms and dads chant rhythmically, like Native Americans doing a rain dance (*Hey . . . ho, ho, ho*), and others imitate the sound of foghorns. Here's how some parents used white noise to guide their babies to serenity:

> Patrick noticed that his baby son, Chance, was calmed by the sounds of aquarium pumps. So he mounted one on each side of his little boy's crib. The noise and vibration helped Chance settle himself and fall asleep.

> "When Talia began screaming in the supermarket, I put my face right next to her ear and uttered a rough *shhhh* until she calmed. While this seemed rude to the people watching me, it soothed her in seconds.
>
> "Once, when Talia had a mini-meltdown at the local FedEx office, I quieted her with this same technique. The shushing worked so well that a clerk asked me for a repeat demonstration, sharing that her daughter had twins and was dying to find a way to relieve their crying."
>
> Sandra and Eric, parents of Talia and Daniel

> "We turned the radio on for our fussy daughter, Camille, but rather than playing soft music, we tuned it to loud hissing static between stations. We noticed that Camille didn't like the popping, crackly sound of static on the AM radio—she was an FM static aficionado! Within a few minutes of tuning in to her favor-

ite nonstation, her face would soften and she'd drift into a peaceful sleep."

Hylda and Hugo, parents of Camille

Steve and Stefanie's six-week-old, Charlie, would only calm in the car if they played a CD with hair dryer sounds during the drive. After he passed four months he was suddenly able to tolerate car rides without the CD noise.

11

~~~~

4th *S*: Swinging—
Moving in Rhythm
with Your Baby

- Why swinging makes babies so happy.
- The three keys to successful motion.
- *Never shake your baby!* How crying and frustration can lead to tragedy.
- Good move: The *Jell-O head* jiggle, *windshield wiper,* and infant swing.
- Tips for getting the most out of your swing.
- Lullabies: What swinging sounds like when it's put to music.

> *Life was so rich within the womb. Rich in noises and sounds. But mostly there was movement. Continuous movement. When the mother sits, stands, walks, turns— movement, movement, movement.*
>
> Frederick Leboyer, *Loving Hands*

Every night, Ellyn and Harold put their colicky baby, Zachary, into his stroller and rolled him back and forth over a low wooden threshold on the floor. With each repetition, Zack got a little jolt, like a car going over a speed bump. Harold would bounce him one hundred times. And if Zach was still fussing after that—he'd do it one hundred more!

Zachary's brother, Nathaniel, preferred another type of motion to quell his yelping. Ellyn held him snugly against her body while "bopping" to the Rolling Stones. She said, "Over four months, we almost wore out our living room carpeting dancing Nathaniel around for hours each night!"

WHY DOES SWINGING MAKE BABIES SO HAPPY?

When we think of the five senses—touch, hearing, vision, smell, taste—we often forget our powerful *sixth* sense. No, not ESP; I'm referring to our ancient and deeply satisfying sense of movement in space. This is the wonderful feeling that gets turned on in a rocking chair or when you sway side to side to settle your infant.

Rhythmic movement, or *swinging,* is a powerful soothing tool. I bet you can remember many times when you were lulled by the hypnotic motion of a swing, hammock, train . . . or *your* mom.

For some babies, motion is the only thing that soothes them. These babies are happiest when *boinged* up and down on the edge of the bed or hippity-hopped around the room. (Slings, swings, and exercise balls are great for these little movers and shakers.)

But why do tiny jiggles relax us so? Because swinging echoes the motion that entranced us inside the womb and turns on the calming reflex.

ONCE UPON A TIME: HOW PARENTS USED SWINGING IN OTHER AGES AND CULTURES

There was something so natural as well as pleasant in the wavy motion of the cradle . . . and so like what children had been used to before they were born.

Michael Underwood, *Treatise on the Diseases of Children*, 1789

Since the dawn of time, perceptive parents have recognized motion's wonderful effect. For our ancient ancestors, soothing babies with continuous movement was easy, because they spent long hours walking with their infants carried on their hips.

Even modern parents find that it's impossible to keep still when holding a baby. You constantly shift your weight, pat her bottom, touch her head, kiss her ears. Imagine how stark the stillness of a bassinet must feel to your baby compared to the gentle strokes and movements that nurture her when she's in your arms.

For most of human existence, placing a baby on the ground was risky . . . so clever parents invented slings and cradles to keep babies protected, free up their mom's hands, and still give calming rhythm.

Gynecology by the physician Soranus is one of the world's oldest medical books (written in AD 200). Some tips from this genius of ancient Rome haven't stood the test of time; for example, he thought carrying a boy on your shoulders could hurt his testicles and turn him into a eunuch. But many of his pearls have proven enduring, such as his recommendation to jiggle babies by "balancing the crib upon diagonally opposed rocks," teetering it back and forth. This idea inspired the invention of the cradle (a crib placed upon rockers instead of rocks) and smart sleepers, which reward babies with a hypnotic, jiggly motion.

In many countries today, babies are still kept in constant motion. They're bounced and wiggled while strapped to the backs of their moms, sisters, or the family yak. Thai parents rock babies in baskets hung from the ceiling. Eastern European moms swing infants in blanket-like hammocks. Persian women sit on the floor, their babies placed in the grooves between their outstretched legs, and pivot their heels side to side, swishing their tiny children like human metronomes.

In the United States, however, parents have long been warned not to handle their babies too much. In the late 1800s, America's leading pediatrician, Dr. Emmett Holt, wrote: "Babies less than six months old should never be played with at all. To avoid overstimulation, babies need peaceful and quiet surroundings." He worried parents would jar their babies' fragile nervous systems. By the 1920s, the question of whether to rock a baby was no longer open to discussion. Quite frankly, no one dared admit to doing it.

In the 1970s, this big myth began to crumble as moms began carrying their babies in slings. Fast-forward to today, and it's obvious that babies *adore* the closeness of being carried. Wearing your baby nurtures her with your warmth, scent, touch, sound . . . and rhythmic jiggles and sways.

In late pregnancy, you may have noticed that your baby got most active when you went to bed (and stopped moving). One mom told me her fetus danced around every night and she would calm him by tapping her bulging belly back and forth, like a woman making a tortilla.

Tiny jiggles calm the fussies much better than slow, broad swinging. Of course, you have to be gentle and always support your baby's head and neck. But in the womb, she was constantly bounced as you walked, hustled up and down the stairs, or salsa'd your way through Zumba classes.

PUTTING THE MOVES ON: USING MOTION TO CALM THE FUSSIES

When Savannah was in the middle of a meltdown, Steve and Cherie would cuddle their four-week-old, sit at the edge of the bed—feet on the ground—and bounce in quick, jerky little motions.

Babies love jiggly motion. Maybe that's why we call infants *bouncing baby girls and boys*! Over the centuries, parents have invented countless ways to move their unhappy infants from tears to tranquility. Here are the top ten:

1. Baby slings
2. Dancing (with quick little moves up and down)
3. Rhythmic pats on the back or bottom
4. Bouncing on the edge of the bed
5. Rocking in a rocking chair
6. Car rides
7. Infant swings
8. Bouncing on an exercise ball
9. Brisk walks
10. Jiggly smart sleepers

A Bonus Eleventh Technique: The Milk Shake

Most parents are amazed how well this method works.

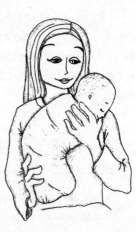

1. Sit with your baby on your lap.
2. Place one hand under your baby's chin like a helmet strap and slip the other under the buttocks.
3. Lean your baby forward—his head a few inches in front of his body—and lift him straight up—a foot or so—into the air.
4. Now, bounce him up and down with

fast (two to three times a second), tiny (one- to two-inch)
movements, like you're making a milk shake.

This is also a great way to burp your baby—and tone your arms.

SWINGING RULES: THE THREE KEYS TO SUCCESSFUL MOTION

> *Those who find that rhythmic rocking doesn't work are*
> *almost certainly rocking too slowly.*
>
> Penelope Leach, *Your Baby and Child*

For fussy babies, the swaddle must be snug, the *shhhhing* strong, and
the swinging bouncy! The rules of successful swinging are:

1. *Start out fast and jiggly.*

   Fussy babies calm best with small, trembly moves . . .
   never more than one or two inches from side to side. This
   jiggling switches on the calming reflex.

   Some babies also like the *free fall* feeling they get when
   their parent dances around and suddenly dips or bends over.
   But if you have a sensitive baby, that motion may upset him
   even more.

2. *Let the head jiggle more than the body.*

   Tiny moves activate motion detectors in your baby's
   inner ear. That's why the movement of the *head*—not the
   body—works.

   Note: Keep your hands a little open so the head quivers,
   like Jell-O on a plate. Holding the head too snugly prevents
   the wiggling needed to flip on the calming reflex.

3. *Follow your baby's lead.*

   Your vigor (of motion) should reflect your baby's vigor
   (of crying). Gentle movements are fantastic for relaxed,

sleepy infants, but the more agitated your baby is, the faster, smaller, and more jiggly you need to be. (The calmer he gets, the slower your swinging can be.)

Jovo and Mina realized they had to play "follow the leader" with their baby: "The most effective way to quiet Mane was putting him on our shoulders and thumping his back . . . fast and firmly. As he calmed, we downshifted the intensity of our pats, bit by bit."

Thumping your baby like a little drum may sound excessive, but most babies love it . . . and it can also help them burp!

IS JIGGLING EVER BAD FOR BABIES?

Ken and Lisa were hesitant to jiggle baby Emily. They were concerned that it would make her spit up, get overstimulated, or even jostle her brain. But when they tried it, they were amazed: "We worried it would be too strong, but it worked like a charm!"

After having a couple of kids, moms learn that fussy babies settle fastest when they're bounced. And fast jiggling is certainly safer than driving around town with a weary dad behind the wheel.

However, many first-time moms and dads find this motion a bit counterintuitive and too intense. "I know it's been done for thousands of years, but is there any risk jiggling can accidentally cause shaken baby syndrome?" Fortunately, the answer is . . . No! No! No!

There's a *huge* difference between shaking and swinging. Shaking is rough and very violent. It bangs the brain back and forth against the hard inner walls of the skull, tearing open tiny veins, causing bleeding and brain damage.

A report by the AAP noted, "The act of shaking leading to

Shaken Baby Syndrome is so violent that individuals observing it would recognize it as dangerous and likely to kill the child."

Swinging, on the other hand, is safe because:

1. The motions are fast but tiny; just one to two inches, side to side. So the brain barely moves at all.
2. The baby's head and neck are always supported and in line with the body. (There is no whipping action with the body going one way and the head flailing abruptly the other way.)

NEVER SHAKE YOUR BABY: CRYING, FRUSTRATION, AND ABUSE

Frank felt anger blow across him like a hot wind. After weeks of his son's colicky screaming, he got so angry he punched his hand right through the door. "I was just so frustrated and exhausted," he said, almost breaking down. "I'd never hurt my boy, but for the first time in my life I understood how a parent could be driven to such desperation."

When you're tired and stressed, your baby's nonstop shrieks can trigger an internal red alert, making your heart pound and your nervous system jump. And if you're already feeling crushed by exhaustion, money stress, and family fights . . . feeling incapable of soothing your baby's screams can push even loving parents into panic, anger, and the dark abyss of child abuse. This happened just outside of Boston in 2010:

Paramedics responding to a 911 call arrived to find a father holding his blue, limp six-month-old. The man, a thirty-one-year-old employee of one of the nation's top universities, said he had been trying to calm his baby's cries by vigorously moving him.

Tragically, the damage to the child's brain was so severe the baby died. The man was put on trial for shaking his baby to death.

Shaken baby syndrome (SBS), also known as abusive head trauma, affects over one thousand babies each year. (A University of North Carolina study estimated that the incidence may even be one hundred times higher!) The average age of the victims is three months. Twenty-five percent die, and survivors usually suffer permanent brain damage.

Several reports have identified crying as the key trigger. A Dutch study discovered that one in twenty parents slapped or shook their baby because of crying. An Estonian study reported that—well before the attack occurred—parents usually contacted their baby's doctor seeking help calming excessive crying.

Today, swinging and the 5 S's are taught in public health programs to *prevent* abuse. Tiny jiggles are perfectly safe! And, they calm babies so quickly they may keep parents from reaching the boiling point of abusive desperation.

Bottom line: Never shake (or even jiggle) your baby when you're angry! If you're at the end of your patience, put your baby down and take a break (even if your baby is crying). Yell into a pillow or punch the sofa if you need to vent your stress, then call for help from your spouse, family, a friend, or a crisis hotline. The National Child Abuse Hotline, 1-800-4-A-CHILD (1-800-422-4453) is open all day, every day.

Kristi Calms Kyle's Colic with the "Jell-O Head" Jiggle

Kristi and John just couldn't figure Kyle out. One night, their copper-haired baby would be fine, but the next he'd scream for hours. Kristi finally called for help after her five-week-old had been shrieking at the top of his lungs for hours.

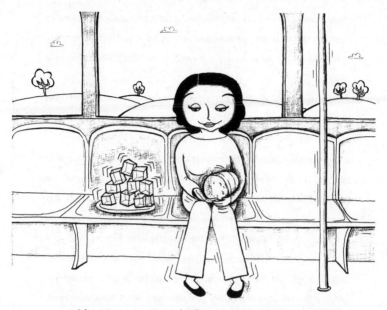

CALMiNG A BABY WiTH THE "JELL-O HEAD" JiGGLE

She describes what happened that Sunday night when the doctor made a house call:

As luck would have it, Kyle finally fell asleep moments before the doorbell rang. I was so afraid the doctor would wake him up, I almost asked him to leave. Sure enough, as soon as he placed his cold stethoscope on Kyle's chest, the shrieking started again.

Apologizing for waking him up, the doctor reassured us that Kyle was a healthy baby who just had trouble self-calming. He swaddled and jiggled our frantic baby, and we were stunned that within a minute Kyle was resting angelically on his lap . . . as if his last explosion had never happened.

John, my mom, and I all practiced the technique in front of the doctor, but when it was time to put Kyle back in his bed . . . we wimped out and asked him to do it one more time before he left. Our boy did great that night, but the next day was terrible again.

Thank goodness, my mom came to the rescue. She wrapped

Kyle, placed him on her lap, *shhhhed* loudly, and did what I came to call the "Jell-O head." Wiggling her knees back and forth, she made his head quiver between her loosely cupped hands, like Jell-O on a plate.

At first, Kyle resisted her efforts, straining against the blanket and crying even harder. But, after three or four minutes he quieted, and after eight minutes he was fast asleep!

My mom repeated this miracle many times during her stay with us, and I began to view her as the baby calming expert. I had a hard time getting the hang of the "Jell-O head," but I eventually got more confident. By the time Kyle was seven weeks old, I could guide him from shriek to smile in less than two minutes flat.

I observed that gentle rhythms helped Kyle when he was already quiet, but he needed big-time jiggling to calm screaming. After a few minutes of motion, he'd sigh with relief. Tension seemed to leave his body . . . and I felt like a great mom!

Kristi and John, parents of Kyle and Cassandra

GOOD MOVE: THE *WINDSHIELD WIPER* AND INFANT SWINGS

Deborah's two-month-old son, Max, loved being lifted up and down, over and over. His poor, tired mom felt like a carnival ride.

Genevieve's mom had to walk her baby, lap after lap, around the block to keep her happy.

Carrying your baby is one of the sweetest treats of being a new mom, but by the end of the day, it can leave you exhausted. How can you jiggle your baby without wearing out your back, your carpet, or your sense of humor?

Here are two user-friendly techniques . . . the *windshield wiper* (great for calming frantic babies) and the infant swing (keeps babies quiet *after* they've been calmed).

Windshield Wiper: Using Your Lap to Quiet Your Baby

The *windshield wiper* combines all the 5 S's for a perfect soothing experience. It's one of my favorite ways of switching on the calming reflex.

Here's what to do:

1. Swaddle your baby (1st S), then sit in a comfy chair with your knees touching and your feet flat on the floor, shoulder distance apart. Sitting forward works best.
2. Place your baby on his side . . . in the groove between your legs (2nd S). His cheek and head will be in your palm and outstretched fingers, on top of your knees, and his ankles on your hip.
3. Slide your other hand under his head so your two hands overlap and his head is cradled in a loose, open grasp.

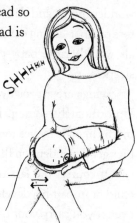

4. Roll him toward his stomach, soften your shoulders, take a deep breath, and let your body relax.
5. Lean over his body and *shhhh* by his ear (the 3rd S). Shush as loud as he's crying.
6. Now, swing your knees side to side—like a windshield wiper (4th S). If he's crying, make faster (two to three beats per second) smaller moves (one inch from side to side) and open your hands to let his head jiggle, like Jell-O.
7. Finally, offer a pacifier (5th S).

Note: The *windshield wiper* motion actually comes from the feet . . . not from your shoulders or hips. Bouncing your knees up and down doesn't work as well as swinging side to side.

Don't get discouraged if the movement seems complicated. You'll soon see it's one of the easiest ways to soothe your baby when you're feeling totally pooped. (It's hard learning anything when someone is yelling at you! So practice the *windshield wiper* when your baby is already calm or sleeping.)

Infant Swings: Get Your Baby into the Swing of Things

Betsy found the swing helpful, but she was so afraid it would hurt Hannah that she put two pounds of bananas in it with her . . . just to slow the thing down!

Many of us live far from our families and the burden of baby care falls on our weary shoulders twenty-four hours a day. No wonder moms and dads need help! So it was inevitable that inventors of labor-saving devices such as dishwashers and garbage disposals would create baby-calming devices such as swings and smart sleepers.

Swings are especially helpful if you have a motion-loving baby. Unfortunately, some parents don't use them because they believe myths like "It moves too fast," "It can hurt a baby's back," or "Babies get dependent on them."

Of course, the last thing you would ever want is to hurt your child or impair his development. But swings are perfectly safe. And even if you carry your baby all day, what happens when you need a break? Without kith and kin to lend support, a swing can help replace a missing pair of hands so you can shower, prepare dinner, or take a nap.

Tips to Get the Most Out of Your Swing

Fern boasted, "The swing became my third hand for little William. The motion worked like magic to get him into peaceful sleep."

There are tricks to getting the most out of your swing:

1. Don't put your baby in a swing when he's screaming. Swings often fail to calm babies mid-meltdown. Try settling your child for a minute or two before using the swing. (Karp's Law of Swings states: If you put a screaming baby in a swing, what you'll get is a swinging, screaming baby!)
2. Swaddle. Snug wrapping helps swinging infants quiet faster and stay quiet longer. Strap your baby securely into the swing's seat *with the bar or belt between his wrapped legs.*
3. Recline the seat *as much as possible.* Sitting up too straight (in a swing, infant seat, or car seat) is not a safe position for a small baby. Their heavy heads can roll forward, kinking the neck, and making it hard to breathe. During the early months, only use a swing that reclines *all the way back* (almost to lying down). Always ask your doctor if your baby is old enough to use the swing.
4. Use white noise. Rumbly sound helps swinging work even better.
5. Use the fast speed. For most fussy babies, the slow speed just doesn't turn on the calming reflex.
6. The twenty-second jiggle. If your swaddled baby starts fussing in the swing, grab the back of the seat and quickly jiggle it . . . just an inch, back and forth. Within twenty seconds, he should relax again. (If not, take him out to see what he needs.)

LULLABIES: WHAT SWINGING SOUNDS LIKE . . . WHEN IT'S PUT TO MUSIC

The word *lullaby* means "sing to sleep." These sweet tunes mimic the reassuring rhythm of a mother's pulse, about seventy beats per second. This pace is perfect for singing—and rocking—your baby as he drifts into the land of Wynken, Blynken, and Nod.

However, soothing songs are often powerless to end crying frenzies. Once in meltdown mode, babies get so lost in their screams they just can't hear us. Just as adults get "blind with rage," babies become "deaf with distress."

Fortunately, many infants can be rescued from their shrieks by switching to a zippier rhythm (two or three beats per second) to catch their attention. If you're a Beatles fan, try jiggling your little fusser to "It's Been a Hard Day's Night." As he settles, slow down to "We Can Work It Out" or "All You Need Is Love." And when he's putty in your hands, downshift all the way to "Golden Slumbers" (or the number-one new-parent fave, "I'm So Tired").

The Other Side of Lullabies

Lullabies calm us all—young and old alike. They soothe our jangled nerves and *lull* us into a peaceful trance. But, did you ever notice that they often contain a dash of black humor? Consider the lyrics of the classic lullaby "Rock-a-Bye Baby":

Rock-a-bye baby on the treetop,
when the wind blows the cradle will rock,
when the bough breaks the cradle will fall,
and down will come baby, cradle and all.

Even the most loving parents need to vent some frustration with a chuckle when they're feeling totally sleep deprived. The rhythms may be designed for sleepy babies, but the words are definitely designed for frazzled grown-ups.

The Whys About the S's: Questions Parents Ask About Swinging

1. *Are swings ever bad for a baby's hips or back?*

   No. In the womb, babies are twisted like pretzels. Their supple bodies are incredibly flexible, which is why they can be placed in a swing with no concern about the back. And, by placing a strap between your baby's legs, you're opening the legs, which is actually a healthy hip position!

2. *Do swings make parents neglect their babies?*

   Of course, you should gift your baby with hours and hours of cuddling. But unless you have a dozen relatives to help, there may not always be enough arms to go around when you have pressing tasks you need to accomplish. That's when swings come to the rescue.

3. *Should I avoid rocking my baby vigorously right after a feeding?*

   Jiggling doesn't make babies spit up more. In fact, by reducing crying, it will help your baby throw up less! Bouncing can also loosen a gas bubble and help your baby burp.

4. *Can a baby get dizzy or nauseous from jiggling?*

   No. Jiggling does not set off the nausea center of the brain. Dizziness and nausea are triggered by big, wide movements such as driving your car down a curvy mountain road. Swinging makes fussy babies feel more comfortable, not less.

5. *If I use the swing too much, will it lose its effectiveness?*

   Some babies love to suck, some need white noise to stay calm, and others are only happy when they're in a sling or swinging all day. Luckily, what babies love, they love all the time. That's why they never tire of milk, cuddling, or swings.

6. *What should I do if my baby cries more when I rock him fast?*

It can take a little time for your infant to realize you're doing something he likes. If he's still yelling thirty seconds after you begin jiggling, check your technique. Make sure your moves are fast and tiny, you're supporting his head and neck, and your hands are open to allow his head to jiggle . . . and don't forget the loud white noise.

A PARENT'S PERSPECTIVE: TESTIMONIALS FROM THE TRENCHES

Here are a few parents whose babies calmed once they got a little mojo happening:

When baby Hudson began to cry, David tried burping him by hoisting his little son onto his shoulder and lightly patting his back. But despite David's loving attempts, Hudson continued to wail.

Perhaps out of frustration—or from some ancient instinct—David started patting him harder. He thumped him like a little tom-tom drum, with a cupped hand, at about two pats per second. Almost instantly, Hudson quieted. His body melted into his dad's arms and a few minutes later he fell asleep. "I was surprised to see how firmly he liked to be patted," said David. "But he relaxed so fast and so deeply, I knew it was right."

When Margie and Barbara's son, Michael, was six weeks old, he screamed so loudly at night that their downstairs neighbor would bang on the ceiling. Margie tried to placate him with gentle rocking and soothing songs, but nothing worked until she discovered what she called the "ancient war dance."

Clutching Michael to her chest—his stomach pressed against her and her arms around him like a straitjacket—Margie loudly chanted, "HA ja ja ja, HA ja ja ja." With each accented "HA" she doubled over and bent at the knees, making Michael feel as if he'd fallen through a trapdoor. With each "ja" she ratcheted her body partway back up. By the third "ja" she was standing straight again, ready for the next "HA."

Margie said that the vigor of the rhythm and the loudness of the chant were the keys to success. Usually Michael was snoozing again within minutes.

Sandy could calm Harriet in her lap, but when she moved the baby to the swing, her little girl roared all over again. Sandy's doctor—and her mother-in-law—warned her not to overstimulate her child, so she always set the swing on the slowest speed.

But it turned out that this was too gentle for her little firecracker. As soon as Sandy began wrapping Harriet snugly, turning on the hair dryer, and quickly jiggling the swing by hand for a few seconds; soothing Harriet became a snap, and the swing began to work every time.

12

<p align="center">~~~~~~</p>

5th *S*: Sucking—
The Icing on the Cake

> *Suck, and be satisfied.*
>
> Isaiah 66:11

Your baby's survival depends on her ability to suck. In fact, this skill is so important that babies start practicing long before birth!

In the womb it's easy for babies to suck their fingers because the soft walls deflect their hands right back toward the mouth. During the fourth trimester, however, your baby won't spend much time sucking her fingers. It's not that she doesn't want to—she'd probably slurp them all day long if she could—but popping a finger in the mouth and keeping it there is a Herculean accomplishment for a newborn. Even when your baby concentrates, her poor muscle coordination makes it more likely that her hands will whack her nose than find her mouth. That's why babies are so relieved when we pop a breast, bottle, or pacifier right into place.

Note: By the time your baby reaches four months she'll be able to park her thumb in her mouth anytime she wants.

SUCKING: INSTANT HAPPINESS

New babies grow so fast they need a milky meal eight to twelve times a day. Some people say they eat like "little pigs," but piglets can't hold a candle to our babies! Every day, our little ones "snort down" three ounces of milk for every pound of their body weight. That's like you guzzling five gallons of whole milk every day, seven days a week!

The wonderful 5th *S* feels extraordinary because it can both satisfy hunger and turn on the calming reflex. All this sucking means hours of pleasure throughout the day.

Some babies will suck anything put in their mouths, but others are little gourmets. Two-month-old Liam refused to suck on anything—not pacifiers, not his fingers, not even a bottle—with one exception: He loved sucking on his mother's upside-down second finger!

Doctors call infant eating *nutritive* sucking and call pacifier use *nonnutritive* sucking (because it yields no nutrition). Non-nutritive sucking helps babies stay calm amid the chaos of the world around them. Like baby meditation, paci sucking lowers the heart rate, blood pressure, and stress levels; it even reduces crying after shots and blood tests. But as hunger builds, your baby will eventually spit the pacifier out, as if to complain, "Hey, I ordered milk—not rubber!"

(After some great *nutritive* sucking—that is, a good feeding—she'll happily accept the binky again.)

Note: As a special bonus, scientists have discovered that sucking a paci at bedtime can lower your baby's risk of SIDS . . . even if she spits it out after falling asleep. (Although doctors have yet to figure out how this bit of sucking works such wonders.)

Can My Baby Suck Too Much?

Some experts warn parents not to let babies suck "too much," saying it's *habit forming*. Fortunately, it's impossible for babies to suck too much. Sucking isn't candy or an addiction; it's an integral part of the fourth trimester and one of your baby's first steps toward self-reliance.

ONCE UPON A TIME: HOW PARENTS USED SUCKING IN OTHER AGES AND CULTURES

One of the sweetest moments of motherhood is when your baby gently drifts into sleep sucking at your breast or on a bottle.

Milk is the center of an infant's world—which is why some people refer to women who breast-feed as *Earth Mothers*. But a more appropriate name for these moms would be *Galactic Goddesses* because the words *galaxy* (and *galactic*) come from the ancient Greek word *gala*, meaning "milk." Legend has it that all the stars in the sky came from milk sprayed out of the breasts of the goddess Juno. Hence, we call our galaxy the Milky Way!

From the Efé of central Africa to the !Kung San tribe of Botswana, moms use sucking as the "go-to" remedy for fussing. At the least little squawk, they bring their babies to the boob thirty . . . forty . . . even *one hundred* times a day!

Besides the breast, inventive moms throughout history have used other sucking solutions to soothe crying. Some let their babies slurp on a bit of sugar enveloped in a little rag. Others upped the ante by dunking this "sugar teat" in brandy. In centuries past, Russian mothers, unable to afford sugar, offered their colicky babies a small piece of chewed-up bread wrapped in a thin cloth.

As rubber bottle nipples became popular in the early 1900s, so did rubber pacifiers. The English called these *dummies* because they helped quiet a baby so quickly. (Similarly, we describe someone unable to hear and speak as *deaf and dumb*.)

HELPING YOUR BABY "SUCK-CEED" WITH PACIFIERS

For many babies, sucking is the most calming of the 5 *S*'s. As just mentioned, in many societies, babies are actually expected to suckle at the breast *dozens of times a day*. In our culture, however, such frequent nursing may not be practical.

To replace all this nursing, some parents are told to teach their babies to "self-soothe" by sucking their thumbs. But finger sucking is difficult for most infants. Like trying to pick up ice with chopsticks, the fingers keeps slipping away despite the baby's best efforts.

Luckily, besides the breast, we have a tool for babies who want to suck all day—pacifiers. Here are a few tips to help boost your baby's pacifier "suck-cess":

- Pick the right nipple. Should you use stubby, little pacifiers with short stems or ones with long stems and tips that are flattened on one side? Ultimately, the perfect pacifier is the one your baby likes the best.
- Don't try the hard sell. Pushing a paci into your baby's mouth when she's crying is often doomed to fail. Try calming her first with the other *S*'s, then as she settles, offer the pacifier.

• Use *reverse psychology*. This is the best trick for teaching your baby how to keep a pacifier in her mouth. It is based on a simple principle: *If it's in my mouth it belongs to me!*

Here's what to do: Offer your baby a pacifier when your little one is calm. Then, when she starts to suck on it, *lightly tug it back* . . . as if you're starting to take it out. (Don't pull so hard that it actually comes out.) After a few times your baby will resist these little pulls . . . and suck harder.

Before you know it, your yanks will feel like trying to pry a toy out of the grasp of a two-year-old; the harder you pull, the more she'll resist! After a week of practice, your baby will probably be able to keep the pacifier in her mouth as long as she wants.

PACIFIER PITFALLS

Hannah thought her son, Felix, was a pacifier addict. "He was hooked on it for years. So, with my second child, I vowed not to use it. Within a few months, however, I caved in because Harmon was so miserable without it . . . and so content with it. I just couldn't deny him that pleasure."

Some folks worry that soothers teach "bad habits." But truthfully, they're just calming tools. Having said that, there are a few paci problems to avoid:

1. **NIPPLE CONFUSION:** Most babies suck anything put in their mouths. But nursing babies sometimes get "confused" if given bottles or pacifiers *before* breast-feeding is going well.

2. **CHEMICALS:** Buy transparent silicone instead of dull, yellow pacifiers. After a while, yellow rubber may deteriorate and release tiny bits of unwanted chemical.

3. **KEEP SWEETS AWAY:** Never dip the paci into syrup. Sweeten-

ers such as honey, maple syrup, or corn syrup can trigger baby botulism (causing temporary paralysis, and even death.)

4. **KEEP IT CLEAN:** When you buy a pacifier, wash it well with soap and hot water. Rinse it when it falls on the floor. Since saliva can carry germs such as cold viruses or herpes, I recommend you not suck on it as a method of cleaning. Interestingly, Swedish doctors found babies grew up to have a little less asthma and eczema if their parents sucked the pacifier to clean it. But your baby's immune system is fragile during the early months of life, so I'd recommend using water to clean it during the fourth trimester.

5. **NO STRINGS ATTACHED:** Never hang a pacifier around your baby's neck. Strings or ribbons may wrap around the throat, creating a choking hazard, or get caught around the fingers, cutting off the circulation.

6. **TIME'S UP?:** Don't worry if your five-month-old still loves the paci. Sucking is wonderfully calming and will help your baby deal with all the crazy, unpredictable new things she encounters every day.

Breast, Pacifier, Thumb: Are You a Family of Suckers?

Some babies soothe with sound, some love motion, and others bliss out sucking the breast or pacifier. This incredible drive to suck is usually just an inherited trait, like eye color or dimples. Or, put another way, sucking is one thing you really *can* blame on your mom!

In my experience, most babies who *love* to suck have a parent (or close relative) who was a dedicated thumb or paci sucker or who had a self-soothing love affair with a blankie or stuffed animal (*lovey*). I've even seen babies with strange sucking preferences—like slurping on two fingers, held upside down—in exactly the same way their moms did it thirty years before!

Sucking can reduce the discomfort of teething and keep your little one calm even in a busy, noisy household.

So don't worry if the paci is your baby's fave stress reducer and she resists your attempts to take it away. If you insist on removing her beloved binky she'll probably just switch to her thumb, which is a much bigger problem! It's almost impossible to wean thumb sucking until your baby decides to stop on her own (which may take many years). Furthermore, finger sucking is more likely to cause serious orthodontic and speech problems, like an overbite or high palate with displaced, crowded teeth.

Real Nipple vs. Rubber: It's Not Nice to Fool a Baby

Nipple confusion happens because sucking on a rubber teat requires a very different mouth and jaw action than sucking on a real nipple. When babies breast-feed they relax and open the mouth wide. Next, they pull the milk out with gentle peristalsis (a wave of muscular contraction passing from the tip to the back of the tongue). Bottle-fed babies, on the other hand, open the mouths less widely and tend to bite the nipple, between the gums, to promote the flow of formula. (You can imagine how that feels on your nipple!)

It's best to avoid all bottles and pacifiers until the nursing is going well. (Although it's no catastrophe if your baby gets a pacifier a few times in the hospital.) Once your baby has the hang of nursing, I recommend giving *one* bottle feeding a day (preferably of breast milk or—if you don't have enough milk pumped—breast plus some warm water that you previously boiled). This way, your baby will learn how to take a bottle from another caregiver, in case you get sick, become unavailable, or have to return to work.

Note: If you wait longer than four weeks to introduce the bottle, you may be rudely surprised by your baby's emphatic *rejection* of the rubber nipple! Once you start bottles, try not to skip more than one or two days without giving one. Some babies stubbornly refuse the bottle if their moms take too long a break. And don't dilute the milk more than once a day. Frequent watered-down feedings are bad for her health.

The Whys About the S's: Questions Parents Ask About Sucking

1. *How can I tell if my baby needs milk or just wants to suck?*

    Look for these signs to indicate that your baby is crying for food:
    - When you touch her face, she turns her head and opens her mouth in search of the nipple.
    - A pacifier initially calms her, but she soon starts fussing again.
    - When you offer her milk she takes it eagerly and after the meal becomes peaceful or sleepy.

2. *Can using a pacifier ever prevent breast-feeding problems?*

    An Oregon State University study found that moms who gave their newborns pacifiers were actually *more* successful at breast-feeding! That's because exhausted moms who were not allowed to give pacifiers to their breast-feeding babies ended up giving formula to soothe the fussing and hunger.

    Once nursing is going well, pacis may also make nursing *more* successful. They give moms a break from the crying and allow other caregivers to soothe the baby. Nevertheless, in general, it's best to avoid pacifiers for the first couple of weeks, if you can.

3. *Can pacifiers cause ear infections?*

    Sucking hard can disturb the pressure in the ears and lead to infections (much the way that kids get ear infections after pressure changes on airplane flights). Fortunately, you don't have to worry about sucking related ear infections for the first six to nine months because young infants usually don't suck hard enough to create much pressure.

4. *Can pacifiers prevent SIDS?*

Studies consistently show less SIDS among infants who get bedtime pacifiers (reducing the risk by about 50 percent)! For this reason, the AAP recommends pacifiers be part of every baby's nap and bedtime routine. (Bottle-fed babies can start from birth; breast-fed babies as soon as the nursing is going well.)

5. *Can my baby get addicted to the pacifier if she always sleeps with one?*

No! That's one myth you can *put to bed*. By weaning it around six or seven months of age, you can reduce pacifier use from many times a day to nothing, in less than a week. However, after nine months, babies often develop emotional attachments to their binky. You can still wean after that age, but be prepared for more protests.

6. *If sucking is so important, should I unwrap my baby's hands so she can get to them?*

No. For the first three months, babies have trouble finger sucking without accidentally hitting themselves in the face. Instead, swaddle your fussy baby and offer your breast or a pacifier. She'll suck better when her arms are not flailing and disturbing her. (If the paci keeps popping out, you can quickly train her to hold it better by using *reverse psychology*, discussed on page 176.)

7. *Will frequent feeding spoil my baby or make her colicky?*

Frequent sucking doesn't lead to spoiling or gas. Studies of native cultures, such as the !Kung San, show that babies were "originally designed" to nurse fifty to one hundred times a day. Yet, !Kung babies don't get gas pains, and their parents rarely need more than a minute to calm their cries.

8. *If I let my baby suckle on my breasts all night, I sleep well and it feels very cozy. But is this okay to do?*

Parents have slept with their babies since the beginning of time. In fact, one of the most delicious feelings a woman can experience is having her sweet baby sleep at her breast. In fact, it is so comforting that tired moms often fall asleep nursing, too! *And, unfortunately, that's where it becomes risky.*

A study of more than two thousand breast-feeding moms revealed that 72 percent of those who nursed in bed fell sound asleep with their babies. And 44 percent fell sleep while nursing on a sofa or recliner. That's very worrisome because increasing numbers of babies suffocate when sleeping in their parents' bed . . . and there is even a *greater risk* when sleeping on a sofa or chair! (See chapter 15 for a detailed discussion about bed sharing.)

If you insist on bed sharing, there are ways to reduce your baby's risk (see the list of protective steps on page 238). But I would still caution you not to bed share for the first nine to twelve months. Research shows that most new parents are sleep deprived, and when we are exhausted we have the same poor judgment and inattention *as someone who's drunk!*

Video studies show that bed-sharing babies spend two-thirds of the night lying in the riskier side position and have their mouths covered with a sheet or blanket for more than an hour each night. When you're bone weary, you might not realize you're accidentally obstructing your baby's face with a blanket or your arm.

So keep your baby right next to your bed—in a co-sleeper, smart sleeper, or bassinet—but don't sleep together on a sofa or bring her into your bed.

A PARENT'S PERSPECTIVE: TESTIMONIALS FROM THE TRENCHES

Some babies suck only when hungry. But for others, sucking is like a massage, meditation, and hot bath all rolled into one!

Rylan's screams terrified Annie and Michael. His heart problem made extreme exertion dangerous. Ann carried him all day until her back was in such pain that she couldn't stand it any longer. She resisted using a pacifier because she "didn't want to teach Rylan a *bad habit.*" Finally driven to desperation, she gave it a try and bingo! the pacifier was a godsend. "We still had to entertain him, but the binky let me take a break, especially when he was in his swinging bassinet."

Valerie recalled, "Our baby, Christina, would scream so much I had to nurse her all day long! But my husband, David, and my mother worried that I was making her more colicky by feeding so often. And my friends warned me I would spoil her by giving in to her wails."

When Valerie confided this to me, I congratulated her on being able to calm Christina during her fussy periods, and I reassured her that it's impossible to spoil a young baby. However, I worried that Valerie was suckling Christina so much, she was ignoring her other calming tools. So, I suggested that David practice the other *S's* to take some pressure off his wife's shoulders.

David loved the idea and soon became a master at calming Christina with swaddling, shushing, and a little pacifier help. He said, proudly, "I feel smart when I can give my little girl what she needs."

Steven and Kelly's one-month-old bruiser, Ian, loved his paci so much he'd scream every time it fell out. Kelly lamented, "It works great, but we feel like we've become his pacifier slaves. My mom joked that we should just tape it in his mouth. Even kidding about that was terrible, but we were going out of our minds."

When Steven and Kelly called their pediatrician, he taught them about *reverse psychology*. One week later, Kelly called back, saying the paci problem was solved. Within just a few days, Ian's mouth muscles were so well trained he could hold the pacifier as long as he wanted without dropping it.

Kelly said, "It's weird. I thought the best way to keep Ian's pacifier in his mouth was to push it back in. But what worked was doing exactly the opposite!"

13

~~~~~~

The Cuddle Cure:
Finding Your Baby's
Favorite Mix of *S's*

MAIN POINTS

- Next steps if the crying continues . . . despite the 5 *S's*.
- Three keys to *S's* success: Precision, practice, and vigor.
- Why dads are the *kings of calm*.

> *To make no mistake is not in the power of man; but from*
> *their errors and mistakes the wise and good learn wis-*
> *dom for the future.*
>
> Plutarch

It's tempting to think someone who's a good baby calmer just "has a gift." But rather than an innate talent, baby soothing is a skill. When you do several—or all—of the *S's* at the same time you'll usually be able to settle your baby's fussing in minutes . . . or less. (A mom I know called her baby's perfect mix of *S's* the Cuddle Cure.) But, what do you do if the *S's* fail?

WHAT TO DO IF THE CRYING CONTINUES

Many babies need more than two S's to settle a big upset. !Kung moms use a mix of tight holding, rocking, nursing, and repeating, "Uhn-uhn, uhn, uhn," over and over. In Tanzania, moms soothe crying by cuddling their babies while pretending to grind corn (vigorously bending and straightening and humming a rough noise). And in our culture, parents drive around their neighborhoods— hitting every pothole and speed bump they can find—soothing their baby's upset with the loud rumble of the motor and lots of jiggly jolts.

Of course, when your baby fusses you should first check to make sure he's not hungry, wet, or lonely. (Even if he just finished feeding, try offering just a little more to eat.) If feeding, holding, and skin-to-skin contact don't seem to be working, the 5 S's usually do the trick. But if *they* don't help, here are some other things to consider:

1. Does your baby have a little problem? Is your child getting too little milk, or perhaps too much? Is she struggling to

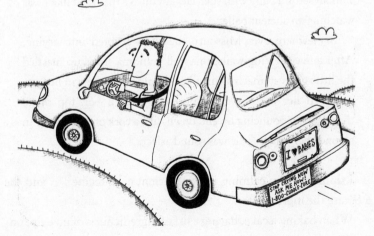

make a poop? Fortunately, little problems like these are usually obvious and easy to resolve.

2. Does your baby have a bigger problem? Five to ten percent of colicky babies have a medical cause of their crying, such as a food intolerance, urinary infection, or stomach acid reflux.

3. Are you doing the *S's* correctly? If the *S's* don't work, nine times out of ten it's either because your frantic baby needs a couple more *S's* or because you need to spiff up your technique a little. So, double check that you are doing the *S's* *exactly right*.

I'll discuss the small and big problems that cause persistent crying in chapter 14 and Appendix A. But since the most common reason the *S's* fail is just a technique issue—such as wrapping too loosely—let's review the three keys to getting your *S's* in gear: precision, practice, and vigor.

PRECISION: IT HELPS TO BE A LITTLE TYPE A

On a plane from New York to Los Angeles, I watched an elderly woman settle a baby with such elegant moves that I felt like I was watching an ancient ballet.

Somewhere over Missouri, the child erupted into crying. After a few piercing wails, this frail grandma stood up, nestled the little girl's stomach against her shoulder, shushed in her ear, thumped her bottom rhythmically, and then—on top of all that—began bouncing up and down, like a cork on the ocean. In seconds her tiny bundle was sound asleep.

I think of baby calming like an ancient cake recipe . . . and the 5 *S's* are the ingredients.

When baking a cake, having a list of ingredients is of no help, unless you also have precise instructions of how much of each ingredient to add, how to grease the pan, what temperature to set the oven, and so forth. If you do each step exactly right you get a perfect cake, but skip steps or do them incorrectly and you end up with warm goop or a blackened, smoking crust!

Unfortunately, most parenting manuals are like incomplete cookbooks. They advise swaddling, rocking, and the like, but don't teach *exactly* how to do each one or how to mix them together. And even when they offer the best techniques, some parents undermine their own success by failing to follow the exact directions or giving up too soon . . . thinking that it just won't work for *their* baby.

But as you now know, reflexes are *all or none* responses. With a knee reflex, whack just hard enough and in the right place and you'll be rewarded with 100 percent success. But, whack too softly—or miss the target by just an inch or two—and you'll get 100 percent failure *even though it looked like you were doing it right*.

Here's a quick recap of the essentials that will help you do each S precisely right:

1st S: Swaddling

Swaddling most often fails when moms abandon it because their babies fight against it. Parents misinterpret their baby's struggling, thinking that it's their baby's way of saying "Let me out! You're unfair!" But, as you now know swaddling is not really meant to calm your baby! Wrapping stops twitches and flailing and allows your baby to regain her composure and focus on the other S's, which *will* turn on the calming reflex.

The best swaddlers make sure:

• The arms are snug and straight at the baby's sides. (The last fold of the *DUDU wrap* goes *across* both arms, holding them down, like a belt.)

- The wrap is loose enough around the legs to allow the hips to bend and the knees to easily open and close.
- The blanket can't easily pop open.
- The baby isn't overheated.

2nd S: Side/Stomach Position

Lying on the back is fine when a baby is calm, and it's the *only* safe position for sleep. But when your baby is fussing, the back is the *worst* position because it can trigger a "red alert" and *amp* up the crying even more. To master the side/stomach position, make sure:

- Your baby is rolled at least a bit toward the stomach. Position-sensitive infants keep crying when they're even *a tiny bit* rolled toward the back.
- Your baby's not hungry. When placed on the side or stomach, a hungry baby's cheek will touch the bedding. That may trigger the rooting reflex, frantically turning his head from side to side, looking for milk. (If your baby roots when turned to the side, offer a feeding before continuing with the S's.)
- Never leave your infant lying on her side or stomach . . . swaddled or not!

3rd S: Shushing

Making a loud "Shhh!" close to your baby's ear can feel totally wrong. Almost like you're saying "Shut up!" This may cause you to hold back and *shhhh* too quietly or too far from your baby's ear. To master this *S*:

- Shush as loud as your baby's cries. Remember, the sound in the womb was louder than a vacuum cleaner.
- Use high-pitch sounds to calm crying and low rumbly

sounds to promote sleep (like the specially engineered high- and low-pitch sounds on the *Happiest Baby* CD/download.)
• Download a smartphone sound meter app to measure the noise level right next to your baby's ear. You'll want 85 to 90 dB of sound for calming crying and around 65 dB to boost sleep.

4th *S*: Swinging

Gentle, slow, wide swings are great to keep calm babies calm, but they're totally ineffective for screamers. To calm those babies:

• Use quick, teensy wiggles (just one to two inches, side to side), two or three times per second.
• Always support your baby's head and neck.
• Hold the head a little loosely in your hands, so it can sort of jiggle . . . like Jell-O on a plate.

Jimmy called me one night; his baby, Jake, was crying loudly in the background. Jimmy told me he tried the *S's,* but they just weren't working. Hearing the concern in his voice, I made a house call and discovered that he was doing everything just fine, except one thing: Rather than quick, tiny moves, he was moving Jake side to side with big twelve-inch swings. Once Jimmy made the moves fast and short—and opened his hands to let Jake's head wiggle a bit—he became the calming master.

5th *S*: Sucking

Sucking is the most natural *S* of all. But if you're having trouble nursing, contact your doctor or the nearest La Leche League group. And if your baby rejects the pacifier, here's how to be a little more persuasive:

- Calm him first. Screaming babies have a hard time latching on.
- Try different brands. Some babies prefer a particular nipple shape over another.
- Use *reverse psychology*. (See page 176.)

PRACTICE: IT DOES MAKES PERFECT

If at first you don't succeed—you're running about average.

M. H. Alderson

Mastering the 5 S's is like learning to ride a bike: strange at first, but lots of fun once you get the hang of it. New abilities are hard to practice when your baby is flailing and yelling at a level that could shatter glass. So start experimenting with the S's when he is already calm or asleep. (You may find that watching *The Happiest Baby* DVD is another way to get totally dialed into these somewhat surprising techniques.)

Before long you will feel much more confident and your baby will calm faster, too. With each repetition of the S's, he'll increasingly recognize what you're doing—and remember how much he likes it.

Note: If you're starting the S's when your baby is past one month old, it may take a few extra days for him to unlearn his prior experiences and become familiar with the new approach. So keep at it and you'll soon be rewarded with success!

VIGOR: DON'T BE OVERLY TIMID!

Jessica tried quieting her frantic six-week-old with swaddling, white noise, and a swing. But, like a little Houdini, Jonathan quickly burst free from the bundling . . . and wailed even harder!

I advised her to straighten his arms, tighten the wrap, crank the swing up to high speed, and switch on a real hair dryer. Those changes led to a big improvement. Soon, Jonathan's daily outbursts shortened from over an hour to under five minutes.

Vigor is the least intuitive, yet one of the most important, element for successful parenting! After all, babies are so delicate that doing *anything* vigorously seems wrong. Breast-feeding, for example, can feel pushy at first. Yet moms who are shy about being assertive often end up with a frustrated baby and sore nipples.

Similarly, most new moms instinctively attempt to calm fussing with *gentle* rocking and *quiet* whispers. But you need some extra oomph in motion and sound to flip on the calming reflex. In fact, the more frantic the cries, the snugger the swaddling, louder the shushing, and the jigglier the swinging must be . . . or they simply won't work.

One mom told me how impossible it was to gently guide her baby from screaming to sleep. "I'm a therapist and I have a lot of practice keeping calm in the face of angry outbursts. I expected my skill at staying balanced would help me guide my one-month-old out of her fits. What a joke! I soon realized that my little brawler absolutely needed me to pick him up and take control of his crying, like police subduing a mob."

Frantic crying calls for spirited, jitterbug-like bouncing and strong, harsh, hissy *sound*. Sobbing requires gentler waltz-paced rocking and shushing. And once your baby relaxes, you can downshift into the hypnotic to-and-fro of slow dancing. (Of course, any bump up in screaming should immediately be met with renewed vigor.)

Note: Newborns are actually *tougher* than we are in a few surprising ways. For example, they can snooze at the noisiest parties and sporting events and scream much louder and longer than we can!

Dads: The Kings of Calm

A nurse in Boise told me about the great baby-calming *chops* of a father she taught in her *Happiest Baby* class.

At a neighborhood softball game, his wife was in the bleachers, their baby on her lap, when all of a sudden the little girl began to wail. The dad immediately called a time-out, sprinted from third base, 5 S'sed his little baby into serenity, and ran back to his position . . . all in under two minutes. The crowd burst into enthusiastic whistling and applause!

To be sure, men are terrible at breast-feeding, but we're quite good at swaddling, jiggling, and shushing. Most of us see wrapping like an engineering task and we're usually pretty willing to add a bit of vigor to our calming. While moms often prefer soft singing and gentle rocking, dads are more comfortable putting enough vigor into the shushing and wiggly jiggling to reach the "takeoff velocity" needed to trigger the *calming*.

THE MORE THE MERRIER: CALMING BABIES WITH MULTIPLE *S'S*

Nina and Dimitri were dismayed that their champion crier, Lexi, got even louder when they used the hair dryer or swing. But they loved discovering that—used together—the hair dryer plus swing worked like a charm.

Just as babies have different hair color, each one differs in the way he needs to be calmed. Some surrender with rocking, some with strong sound, and others settle the moment they're rolled to the stomach. Easy babies just need one or two of the *S*'s to feel calm and serene. Über-cranky kids, on the other hand, need three or four *S's* to cease screaming. And the fussiest babies keep wailing until they get five *S's* . . . all at the same time.

Tune In to Your Baby's Cuddle Cure: An Experiment in Soothing

Find your baby's favorite *S's* by placing her on her back when she's a bit fussy. Then, start adding them—one by one—and see how many it takes to settle her down.

1. *Shhhh* softly. If that doesn't work, do it louder . . . right near to the ear.
2. Swaddle her (to stop the flailing) while continuing to shush (or while playing a white noise CD or download).
3. Place your wrapped baby on her side or stomach and keep on shushing.
4. Add quick, tiny, jiggly motion.
5. Finally, while continuing all of the above, offer your breast, a pacifier, or your finger to suck on.

14

~~~~~

Other Colic Remedies:
From Old Wives' Tales to
Proven Soothers

███ MAIN POINTS ███

- Ancient colic cures: Massage and walking in the fresh air.
- Three medical crying triggers: Allergies, constipation, and feeding problems.
- Dubious colic treatments: Herbs, homeopaths, chiropractors, and osteopaths.

> *Put cotton in your ears and gin in your stomach!*
>
> Nineteenth-century colic advice

Over the centuries, experts have come up with many new colic "cures." Unfortunately, these best guesses only led to a string of dead-end therapies, from whiskey to sedatives to burp drops. However, besides the 5 S's there are a few other "true paths" for reducing colic.

COLIC CURES FROM GRANDMA'S BAG OF TRICKS

Two great, time-honored soothers are massage and walks outside.

Massage: The Miracle of Touch

Massage is love, which is one unique breath, breathing in two.

Frederick Leboyer, *Loving Hands*

There's an old saying, "A child is fed with milk and praise," and I would say a baby is fed with *milk and caresses*. In the womb, babies enjoy a feast of velvety cuddling twenty-four hours a day. Once born, they still love to be carried and stroked. In fact, your skin-to-skin embrace is the touch equivalent of hypnotic womb motion or whooshing.

Touch is much more than a reminder of the womb; like milk, it's an *essential nutrient* for growth. In some ways, touch is even more important than milk. Consider this: Giving your baby extra milk won't make her any healthier, but the more touches and hugs she gets, the stronger and happier she'll become!

A brilliant baby watcher, Tiffany Field, confirmed the enormous benefits of touch in a series of studies of nurses, mothers, and babies. In one experiment, nurses massaged a small group of preemies for fifteen minutes, three times a day, for ten days. Astoundingly, these babies gained 50 percent more weight and were able to go home almost a week earlier than babies who didn't get massage. In an equally impressive follow-up study, massaged babies examined one year later had higher IQs than those who received just routine handling. Dr. Field also found that healthy, full-term babies who were massaged for fifteen minutes a day cried less, gained weight better, were more alert and socially engaged, and had lower levels of stress hormones. And their moms felt calmer and more relaxed, too!

Walk It Off: Baby Calming Can Be a Stroll in the Park

If babies could talk, they'd bug us all the time: *"Pleasssse* can we go outside?" Infants adore hearing the wind in the trees, feeling fresh air on their face, and watching the passing shapes and colors. Our ancient relatives spent most of the day outside, and some people think that modern babies fuss so much because they're deadly bored at home.

Outside walks fit the idea of the fourth trimester because the entrancing flow of sensations lulls babies, like multisensory white noise. Going for a walk may soothe your baby's fussing, lift your spirits, and fill you both with a deep sense of peace.

OTHER COLIC REMEDIES: A DOCTOR'S BAG OF TRICKS

Five to ten percent of colicky babies have a medical reason for their fussiness. The top concerns relate to four different tummy troubles: Food allergies, constipation, eating issues (over- or underfeeding), and stomach acid reflux. These babies may get some relief from massage, walks, and the 5 S's, but what they really need is a solution for their problem.

Food Allergies: Getting Tummies Back on Track

Of all the problems triggering persistent crying, food sensitivity and allergies rank right at the top. Food issues account for about 90 percent of colic *caused by a medical issue.*

Babies suffering from allergies usually fuss throughout the day (not just at night) and have loose stools, sometimes with streaks of bloody mucus. Unfortunately, no simple test has been found to diagnose these problems. Figuring out if your child has a food sensitivity requires you to play Sherlock Holmes and carefully collect clues.

If you're breast-feeding, your doctor may recommend that you go a week without consuming cow's milk, eggs, peanuts, tree nuts, wheat, soy, and fish to see if the crying improves. If you're bottle feeding, she may suggest you try a special *hydrolyzed* formula containing milk proteins that are "predigested" into tiny, non-allergenic fragments. In past decades, we used to recommend switching to soy or lactose-free milk . . . or even a formula based on lamb protein, but there's no evidence that any of these are truly effective for colic.

If you do decide to try dietary changes, keep a daily journal for a week to keep track of any improvement in crying. Any reduction in fussing *may* be proof of an allergy, but it also may be a coincidence. Your baby's doctor should suggest you do a *food challenge* to really figure things out: After avoiding certain foods for a week, reintroduce a spoonful of the suspected food into your diet (if you are nursing) or feed your baby an ounce of the suspected formula. Try it once a day over four days; if there's an allergy, your baby's crying (and/or mucousy stools) will probably return within a day.

Note: Always ask your doctor before altering your baby's diet . . . or your own.

Constipation: Interesting Ideas on a Dry Subject

Like Grandma said, "It's important to stay regular," and that's especially true for babies. Fortunately, breast-fed babies almost never get hard stools. They may skip a few days between poops, but even then, the consistency is pasty to loose. Bottle-fed babies, on the other hand, can get hard stools, but a couple of commonsense ideas can usually correct the problem:

• Change formula. Starting a new formula may resolve constipation. Some infants have softer stools when they drink formula from concentrate versus powder based (or vice versa). Ask your baby's doctor for guidance.

• Slightly dilute the mix. Your baby's poops may improve when you add a tablespoon of organic adult prune juice or one ounce of water into the formula, once or twice a day (never give dilute formula more often than that).

Note: *Never* give honey or corn syrup as a laxative, before the first birthday (see page 199).

• Open the door. Babies trying to poop often have trouble tightening their stomach muscles and relaxing the rectum at the same time. They accidentally clench the anus—when they should be relaxing it—and consequently, they strain to poop! To help "loosen" your baby's anus, bicycle her legs and massage her bottom. If this fails, insert a Vaseline-greased thermometer or cotton swab—just one-half to one inch—into the anus. Babies usually respond by grunting and pushing the object out . . . often pushing out the poop at the same time.

A Poop Advisory: When Is Constipation a Sign of Something Serious?

After the first couple of weeks, babies usually settle into a pretty good pooping routine. For bottle-fed babies, that schedule is about once or twice a day. Breast-fed babies may actually skip a day or two between bowel movements. In fact, by one month of age, they sometimes go a week or two without having a stool!

When should you be concerned? The best rule is to call your baby's doctor if more than three days pass without a stool. *Call even sooner if your baby has a weak cry, weak suck, or is acting ill.*

The doctor may want to do an evaluation for three rare diseases that can masquerade as constipation:

1. Hypothyroidism: A totally curable condition caused by an underactive thyroid gland. If left untreated, hypothyroidism is a serious problem because it may slow mental development.

2. Hirschsprung's disease: This rare problem occurs when the nerves in the rectum don't develop properly. The baby's rectal muscles tightly clench—unable to relax—which blocks the poop from passing and causes an intestinal obstruction. Fortunately, this problem can be corrected with surgery.

3. Infantile botulism: A rare disease in babies under one year of age characterized by the sudden onset of weakness and paralysis. It's caused by botulism spores hiding in liquidy sweets, such as honey or corn syrup. For this reason, these should *never* be given to babies under one year of age.

For more information on medical issues, see Appendix A.

Fretful Feeding—Too Much (or Too Little) of a Good Thing

Fortunately, 99.9 percent of the time, your baby's hunger and your milk supply are in perfect balance. However, nursing moms occasionally get into a cry-causing imbalance with too little milk . . . or too much.

"Got Milk?" Crying from Too Little Milk

It's easy to tell if a bottle-fed baby is getting her fair share: Just count the ounces she eats. With breast-feeders, however, it's trickier. The following questions may help you to figure out if your nursing baby is crying from hunger:

• Do you have enough milk? Your breasts should feel heavy when you wake up. They may occasionally leak and you should be able to hear your baby gulping at least at the beginning of feedings.

- Is your baby serene after a meal? Well-fed babies get blissful and relaxed after a nursing.

- Does your baby pee enough? During the first days, infants don't urinate very often. But once the milk comes in, they pee five to eight times a day, and the urine is clear or light yellow. If you're just seeing a few wet diapers a day and the color of the pee is dark yellow, consider it a *red alert* and call your pediatrician to check for a problem.

- Is your baby gaining enough weight? Moms—and grandmas—often worry that their child is *too* skinny. Babies usually lose eight to twelve ounces over the first few days of life, but thereafter they gain four to seven ounces per week. But there's no need to guess if your infant is gaining enough weight, simply put her on a scale . . . at the doctor's office. (Most home scales are so inaccurate, they'll drive you crazy!)

If you answered "No" to any of these questions, call your baby's doctor to find out if your child's cries are a sign of insufficient milk.

Note: One last way to check for hunger is to offer a bottle of pumped milk or formula to see if your baby quickly gulps it down. But be careful when giving bottles *before* the breast-feeding is well established. It can alter a child's sucking and make her suddenly reject the breast. In fact, to avoid nipple confusion its best to give no more than one bottle a day, even *after* the nursing is well established.

"My D Cup Runneth Over!" Crying from Too Much Milk

At seven weeks, Luca began to struggle with feedings. He had always eaten with gusto, but now after two minutes he'd arch and wail almost as if he hated being in his mom's arms. But as soon as he was put down, he confused his poor parents by crying even harder!

Frustrated and demoralized, his mom wondered if her milk supply had dried up. Actually, Marija had plenty of milk—in fact, she had *too much*. When Luca finished eating—and just wanted to suck for pleasure—Marija's breasts continued spurting fast little streams of milk. Luca literally had to pull away to avoid choking, but he was in a pickle because he still wanted to suck.

Once Marija began holding her nipple like a cigarette—pressing her fingers together—she was able to slow the flow of the milk, and Luca became an easy feeder again.

Some babies love milk so much, they overeat. They guzzle four to eight ounces at a feed—gulping down lots of air at the same time—and then vomit it all up. Other babies gobble not out of gluttony, but out of self-protection. Their mom's milk pours out so fast, they're gulping and sputtering simply trying not to choke.

Flooding can also happen with bottle-feeding. When the rubber nipple is too soft, or the holes in it are too large, infants can gag like they're drinking from a running faucet.

These questions may help you figure out if your flow is too much for your baby:

- Does your milk spray out of one breast when your baby is sucking on the other?
- Does your baby gulp and guzzle loudly?
- Does your infant struggle, cough, or pull away as soon as the milk starts to flow into her mouth?

If you answered *yes* to these questions, try a little experiment to see if the crying stops when you slow the flow: Right before a feed, express one or two ounces out of each breast. Then, holding your nipple between your second and third fingers, like a cigarette, press your fingers inward—toward your ribs—while you feed your baby. Was there less sputtering and struggling? (You can also try nursing lying down—with your baby on top of you—to try to slow the flow.)

HERBS, HOMEOPATHS, CHIROPRACTORS, AND OSTEOPATHS: COLIC CURES OR DEAD ENDS?

Over the past few decades we've been rediscovering the great benefits that can be realized by using integrative medical practices such as acupuncture and mindfulness. What about for colic? Do alternative approaches help?

Herbal Teas: A Cuppa Comfort?

Through the ages, teas to aid digestion have been recommended for unhappy babies. Traditionally, mothers brewed chamomile, peppermint, fennel, or dill for their babies' upset tummies.

The ancient roots of this practice are reflected in the names different cultures have chosen for these herbs. In Spanish, peppermint is called *yerba buena,* meaning the "good grass"; in Serbian it's *nana,* meaning "grandmother." Dill was used to settle stomachs in ancient Egypt and Greece, and in Viking times. Its English name derives from the Old Norse word *dilla,* meaning "to soothe or calm."

Chamomile is said to have calming properties; peppermint may ease intestinal spasms; dill helps soothe gas; and fennel has been reported to dilate intestinal blood vessels, perhaps facilitating digestion.

Interestingly, some studies have shown a lessening in crying after fussy babies are given herbs. An Israeli report found a tea containing chamomile, fennel, vervain, licorice, and balm mint lessened fussing more than placebo. And an Italian study found that drops of chamomile, fennel, and lemon balm extract had some benefit.

In general, I prefer not giving babies *any* oral supplements or remedies, but if you want to try some tea, here's how:

Prepare dill or fennel seeds by crushing some between two spoons or put some in a small bag and mash them a few times with the bottom of a heavy mug. Place two teaspoons of the broken seeds in a cup of boiling water, let it steep for ten minutes, then strain it and let it cool. Offer your baby a teaspoon of this brew several times a day.

Dill is also found in "gripe water," a folk remedy for colic that can be found in stores in the United States, Great Britain, and the Commonwealth nations. This remedy has never been shown to be effective, and it often contains unwanted sugar, sodium bicarbonate, and other additives.

Note: Never give tea made of star anise! It can cause neurological problems, including seizures.

Other Alternative Practices: Are They Worth a Try?

Homeopathy is a philosophy of healing that teaches "like cures like." In other words, the illnesses can be cured by giving a tiny dose of something that—in a large dose—would actually cause the very same problem. For example, a homeopath might recommend minuscule amounts of poison ivy extract to stop an itchy rash.

Some of the homeopathic treatments recommended for colic are chamomile, colocynth, magnesium phosphorica, and pulsatilla. Some parents swear by them, but there is no convincing evidence of benefit. Over $2.5 billion has been spent by the National Institutes of Health to test herbal and other alternative health remedies. Unfortunately, almost no effective homeopathic tonics have been found.

And just because a medicine is labeled homeopathic doesn't mean it is harmless. Two medical reports have detailed how one colic treatment, named Gali-col Baby, was associated with near-death choking reactions in twelve babies.

The same skepticism relating to homeopathy surrounds claims that chiropractic or osteopathy calm crying. These anatomical approaches to colic assume a birth-related skull and/or spinal misalignment. But if birth trauma was the cause of colic, why is it that preemies never have colicky screaming . . . until they reach their due date? And, why does colic spontaneously evaporate after three to four months? Studies have yet to produce clear evidence that bony manipulation reduces infant fussing.

Note: Manipulation of a baby's skull (cranial) bones may be a harmless expense, but I am very concerned that spinal adjustment risks seriously injuring a baby.

The bottom line: Give the 5 S's a good chance to work. If you're not seeing benefit, ask your doctor's advice before using *any* medical or alternative treatment.

15

~~~

The Magical 6th *S*:

Sleep!

MAIN POINTS

- Baby sleep during the fourth trimester.
- A dozen sleep myths: Reasonable ideas . . . that are totally wrong.
- *Wake and sleep:* Why it's smart to wake a sleeping baby.
- Using the 5 *S*'s to help your baby sleep longer and better.
- Easy steps to wean older infants off the 5 *S*'s.
- The truth about putting babies on a schedule.
- SIDS and suffocation: How to prevent this nightmare.
- Co-sleeping: Why room sharing is good, but bed sharing is risky.

At Ally's two-month checkup, her mom told me she only slept for three-hour stretches during the night. Shaya said getting up so often to tend to the baby was making her more impatient with her other two young girls.

I asked if she was still doing swaddling. She wasn't. "I stopped about a month ago because the nights have been so warm and, besides, she always gets out of it!" I suggested she dress Ally in just a diaper, wrap her tightly in a light muslin blanket—big enough to securely tuck completely around her body—and to play rumbly white noise for all naps and nights. The next week, Shaya reported good news. Ally was now sleeping safely, on her back, for almost six hours every night.

Ahhh . . . sleep!

For most new parents, a good night's sleep shimmers in our weary minds like a distant mirage.

The odd thing is that babies actually sleep quite a bit! During the early months, they rack up more snoozing than at any other time of life, averaging sixteen hours a day.

However, between feeding, bathing, diaper changes, and calming crying, it can seem like you never get a break. And, if your little bunny is one of the 10 percent who sleep only fourteen hours per day—or who sleep all day and feed all night—the first months may push you right to the edge.

How long should your baby sleep?

Most newborns sleep fourteen to eighteen hours in a twenty-four-hour period. It's a good amount, but because it's broken into snippets (twenty minutes to four hours long), for tired parents it may feel like getting a thousand dollars—in pennies.

Scientists disagree on whether breast- or formula-fed babies sleep better. Some studies show formula-fed babies wake more often (and their moms sleep less), but other studies show breast-feeders wake the most. And other studies show no difference whatsoever!

Expect to nurse your baby ten to twelve times a day during the first month. But that doesn't mean you will feed every two hours all night long. Once your milk supply is established (usually after a couple of weeks) offering the breast frequently during waking hours will fill your baby up during the day, which will help your baby go longer (three to four hours) between night feedings.

Of course, you'll need to monitor your baby's weight and pay attention to her daily urine output to make sure she's getting enough. (Infrequent, dark yellow urine is a sign of too little milk intake.)

Whether your baby is a breast or bottle feeder, the 5 S's will improve his sleep. And an extra bonus of a bit more shut-eye is that it boosts your milk supply, lowers your risk of mastitis, and reduces postpartum anxiety and depression.

> *Our two-month-old, Julian, will be our last baby, and as crazy as it sounds, I look forward to nursing him in the middle of the night! It's the only time when we can really be alone, and I get to enjoy my delicious little boy in peace and quiet.*
>
> Gretchen, mother of three

Can You Be Asleep and Awake at the Same Time?

We all have cycles of waking and sleep, but did you know they're not really opposites? When we're very tired—but still awake—we have little *micro*sleeps. Parts of the brain are actually asleep, even though we're still walking, talking and functionally awake! (No wonder drowsy drivers get into more car accidents.)

And in sleep you still get a constant stream of information from the world around you. You'll hear the phone ring and rarely fall out of bed, even though you may be perched right on the edge.

Likewise, babies are not totally "out of it" even while they slumber. That's why they wake more often when they're understimulated: Unswaddled . . . in total silence . . . in an unmoving bed.

BABY SLEEP DURING THE FOURTH TRIMESTER

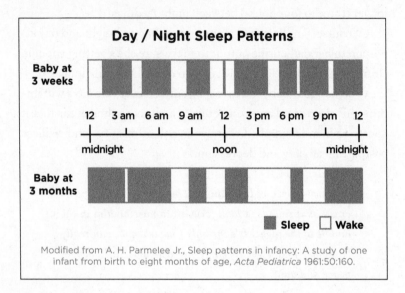

Modified from A. H. Parmelee Jr., Sleep patterns in infancy: A study of one infant from birth to eight months of age, *Acta Pediatrica* 1961:50:160.

As you can see in the sleep graph, three-week-old infants usually sleep in two-, three-, or four-hour blocks (in gray), alternating with hour-long awake times (in white). Two-thirds of each day is spent asleep, but initially the longest stretches of sleep last less than four hours. By three months, awake periods merge into longer clumps, and half of all babies enjoy uninterrupted sleep extending for five hours or more.

As the fourth trimester progresses, your baby will increasingly divide each day into three distinct parts:

- Awake time: For eating and learning about the world.
- Quiet sleep: For resting/recovering from the day's efforts.
- Active (REM) sleep: For dreaming and "reviewing/ remembering" the lessons of the day just past.

As you can see in the graph on page 209, *quiet* sleep makes up 50 percent of a newborn's slumber. In quiet sleep, your baby is "out

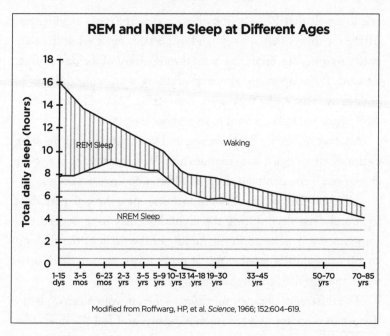

REM and NREM Sleep at Different Ages

Modified from Roffwarg, HP, et al. *Science*, 1966; 152:604–619.

like a light." His breathing is easy and regular; his face still and angelic; but his arm and leg muscles are a little stiff (not floppy like a rag doll's).

The other 50 percent of your baby's snoozing consists of *active* sleep (also called REM—rapid eye movement sleep). It's filled with bursts of brain activity and tiny, jerky eye movements and it occurs between islands of quiet sleep,

REM is the magical time when dreams are spun and memories are filed away. In active sleep your baby's breathing becomes irregular; his arms get as floppy as cooked spaghetti; and little twitches and spectacularly heart-melting grins will come and go. Contrary to myth, these early grins are not a sign of gas. Your baby is trying out what will soon be his most powerful social tool, smiling.

As you can see in the chart, adults get around two hours of active sleep each night. Yet, babies revel in *eight hours* of REM. Why do they clock in so much more than we do? No one knows for sure, but one theory is that REM's "job" is to review the day's experiences, sifting for things that are new and important. Since adult lives are pretty routine, our brains can scan through most of the day on fast-forward. By comparison, almost everything is amazing and new to your baby. That's why they need more REM. "Wow! So much new stuff happened today. I want to remember *everything!*"

Another difference between you and your baby is that his sleep cycles are shorter: just sixty minutes long. Which is why he may wake every hour if you don't use sleep cues like swaddling and sound.

All of us—babies, children, and adults—pass through periods of light and deep sleep during the night. You may have noticed that sometimes you wake up in the middle of the night at the slightest sound or a whiff of smoke. Yet, at other times you are *dead to the world* and can sleep through a ringing telephone!

The difference depends on exactly when in your sleep cycle the disturbance occurs. We arouse most easily, and feel the most alert and refreshed, when we are roused from the lightest levels of sleep, and we feel grumbly and disoriented when we're shaken from the deep, sleepiest part of the cycle.

But, unlike infants, our cycles are closer to ninety minutes long. That may sound like an insignificant difference, but it's exactly why some sensitive babies wake up so often!

Think of it this way: Light and deep sleep cycles repeat all night long, like alternating meat and cheese stacked on a sandwich.

Quiet and active sleep cycles repeat all night long, like alternating meat and cheese stacked on a sandwich. Infants with good state control and mellow temperaments tend to fall right back into slumber even if they wake during light sleep, unless they're uncomfortable or hungry. But infants with poor self-calming and challenging temperaments often wake—and cry—during each cycle of light sleep.

Note: For more tips on boosting sleep between birth and five years of age you might want to take a peek at *The Happiest Baby Guide to Great Sleep.*

A DOZEN SLEEP MYTHS: REASONABLE IDEAS ... THAT ARE TOTALLY WRONG

I'm sometimes amazed by the crazy things people accept as fact. For instance, as recently as the 1960s, doctors said that babies felt no pain during circumcision and that crying was good exercise for a baby's lungs. We even believed that *opium* drops were the best way to relieve colicky crying!

But before you hurt yourself laughing too loudly, you may be surprised how many crazy ideas modern doctors—and parents— believe are true. Here are a dozen of the most common baby sleep *myth-conceptions*!

Myth 1: It takes months for babies to learn to sleep well at night.

No. It usually only takes a few weeks ... if you use the right sleep cues. Your baby just needs you to consistently use swaddling and rumbly white noise—or a smart sleeper—and to practice the *wake-and-sleep* technique every night. (More about that on page 212.)

Myth 2: Sleeping babies need complete quiet.

No. Babies are experts at falling deeply asleep at noisy parties. (Could *you* do that?) In the womb, babies are surrounded by loud, rumbly whooshing twenty-four hours a day. So a quiet room is actually a *sensory desert* to your baby ... sort of like sticking you in a dark closet!

Myth 3: Using rocking or nursing every night to put your baby to sleep will create a dependency on those cues.

Okay, this one's *not* a myth, but it is a myth-conception that dependency is a bad thing!

Let me explain: We all use particular cues to help us relax into sleep. (Do you prefer a dark room? Special pillow? Favorite sheets? Reading? TV? White noise?)

Long before delivery, your baby got used to the calming rhythms he enjoyed every minute of pre-birth slumber. That's why rocking, shushing and cuddling your baby to sleep work so well . . . and why car rides help. But these cues can become problematic because: a) they're very hard to wean (you can't gradually reduce them every day) and b) they slow your baby's learning to self-soothe (the ability to fall back asleep when accidentally awakened).

The good news is that swaddling and white noise (or a smart sleeper's soothing motion) can soothe your baby to sleep *and still* help her learn great self-soothing skills.

Wake-and-Sleep: Why You Should Always Wake a Sleeping Baby

Waking your sleeping baby up every time you place her in the bassinet may sound *crazy,* but it's the best way to help her learn to self-soothe. Here's what you do:

- Prepare: Swaddle your baby, turn on rumbly white noise, and do a feeding.
- Lull to sleep: Let your baby fall asleep in your arms or at the breast.
- Put in bed: Gently slide her into the bassinet or smart sleeper, but once there *wake her* for five to ten seconds (jostle her or tickle/scratch the bottom of her feet).

As long as she's swaddled and shushed and her tummy is filled with milk, she should fall back to sleep quickly . . . with little crying. And during those few seconds—without being held, nursed, or rocked—she will start learning to self-soothe. (You can read more about *wake-and-sleep* at www.happiestbaby.com.)

Note: If your baby resists falling back to sleep, crank up the white noise and jiggle the bassinet for a few seconds. If the crying continues just pick your baby up, soothe her to sleep, and then wake her a little—again—when you place her back down.

Myth 4: Swaddling should be stopped at two months.

Totally wrong! In fact, two months is the *worst* time to stop wrapping your baby! Crying and night waking peak at two to four months. That's exactly why that is a peak time of marital stress, child abuse, postpartum depression, unsafe sleeping practices, breast-feeding difficulties, car accidents, and parental obesity. But swaddling quickly reduces infant fussing and parental exhaustion.

Wrapping also reduces a baby's ability to roll to the stomach. However, if she can roll—despite being swaddled—check that you're wrapping correctly and make sure to use strong, rumbly white noise *all night*. Also, ask your doctor about using a smart sleeper with a special sleep sack to prevent accidental rolling.

Myth 5: Never wake a sleeping baby.

Nope. As just mentioned, you should *always* wake your sleeping baby . . . when you place him down to sleep. The wake-and-sleep technique is the first step in helping your little one develop the ability to self-soothe after a startle or hiccup rouses him in the middle of the night.

Myth 6: Letting babies cry themselves to sleep makes them better sleepers.

Hmmm . . . perhaps. To promote better sleep, most doctors recommend leaving babies alone, to cry in the dark. They advise either not coming back until the morning (the *extinction* sleep training method) or returning every few minutes to give reassurance (the *controlled crying* sleep training method).

But ignoring your baby's nighttime cries goes totally against your parental instincts. Letting your baby scream to "teach her to sleep" is as crazy as ignoring your car alarm while you wait for the battery to go dead. I'll admit that I've used controlled crying on the rare occasions when parents desperately needed some lifesaving sleep, but it really is a last resort.

Fortunately, with the 5 S's or a smart sleeper, most babies can quickly learn good sleep habits without ever being left to cry.

Myth 7: Some babies need their arms out for sleep.

Not really. Parents who notice that their baby stretches the arms up during sleep often assume that their baby needs their arms "free." But that is rarely the case.

We may not want to be swaddled, but for babies, it imitates the cuddly confines of the womb, and it prevents startles and upsets during the night. At first, your baby may resist arms-down wrapping, but with a bit of practice—and a good, rumbly white noise—he'll get used to having his arms in, and sleep much better for the first months of life.

Myth 8: Babies should sleep in their own rooms.

There's no rush to your baby becoming independent. In fact, putting your baby in another room is highly inconvenient for nighttime care and feeding. Plus, room sharing during the first six months has been shown to reduce a baby's risk of SIDS.

Myth 9: By six months most babies sleep through the night.

Actually, this one is wrong on two counts.

First, even by six months, about half of all infants still wake and ask for assistance once a night . . . and babies who bed share wake even more often.

Second, *no baby ever sleeps through the night!* (In fact, neither do older kids or adults.) We all wake—slightly—two to three times a night when we enter the light sleep part of our sleep cycle. If our room has changed since we fell asleep (our pillow fell on the floor, there is smoke, and so forth), we usually wake all the way. However, if everything is as it was when we dozed off, we dive back into slumber so fast we don't even remember waking. Likewise, when your baby lightly awakens, if there's a big change from when she fell asleep (for example, if she's no longer in your arms or at your breast) she'll tend to wake all the way. Fortunately, once she learns self-soothing (with the help of just a little white noise and swaddling), she'll easily fall back to sleep . . . unless she's hungry or uncomfortable.

Myth 10: Babies must adapt to the family, not the family to the baby.

This one is just silly. A key goal of parenting is building your baby's confidence and trust. During the first nine months, creating a sense of security is much more important than pushing her to develop a sense of independence. (You'll have plenty of time in the months ahead to teach limit setting and discipline.)

Myth 11: Keeping babies awake during the day helps them sleep more at night.

Nope. Keeping a tired baby awake usually backfires, leaving him overtired, miserable, and fighting sleep! On the other hand, babies who are to sleep every couple of hours throughout the day are more resilient and fall asleep faster and easier, as long as they're put to bed before they get bleary-eyed and exhausted.

Myth 12: Swaddling is bad for nursing.

Quite the opposite. Some consultants warn moms that swaddling can interfere with nursing. They worry that babies can't give moms early hunger cues—like hands to the mouth—if the arms are straightened and snugly wrapped. Fortunately, this is not a concern. If you miss an early feeding sign, your baby's hunger will just increase a little more and he'll send you other hunger signals—including fussing and crying—within another ten or twenty minutes. In fact, by waiting a little he'll take a bigger, better feeding, instead of snacking all day.

Your Baby's Feeding Signals

Infants have a sophisticated vocabulary for communicating their needs. When mild hunger begins, your baby will show *early* signs, such as putting his hand to his mouth, and making *mmmm* sounds. These signals occur two to three times an hour. (!Kung moms respond to their babies' early cues and nurse fifty to one hundred times a day.)

What happens if you miss an early sign? Don't worry; your baby won't give up. Next, he will send you more demanding middle-hunger cues. These include rooting (moving the head side to side with an open mouth, looking for a nipple), open eyes, and more active movements. If he still hasn't gotten your full attention, he'll shift into late hunger cues: wriggling, fussing, and crying.

Of course, you should never ignore your baby's later signals. In fact, even if your baby fusses ten minutes after the last feeding, you should still offer a bit more milk. (Some babies finish a feeding, but fuss a little later when they realize they need just an extra ounce to "top off the tank" in preparation for sleep.)

But, ignoring *early* signs to get a bit more sleep is actually smart.

An extra hour of rest can improve nursing by reducing depression, preventing mastitis, and boosting your milk supply. That's why hundreds of breast-feeding clinics help nursing moms succeed by teaching them swaddling and the other *S's* during *Happiest Baby* classes.

Note: During the first month or two, you will encourage better nighttime sleeping by waking and nursing your baby every couple of hours . . . *during the day*.

THE BEST SLEEP CUES: BOOSTING SLEEP WITH THE *5 S'S*

We all use special cues to prepare us for sleep. Give me a cool room, feather pillow, firm mattress, rain on the roof white noise—and I'm out like a light. Others fall asleep reading a book or watching TV. I bet you even know some adults who are so "addicted" to two sleep cues—beds and pillows—that they absolutely refuse to stay at hotels that don't have them!

Okay, you get my point: We're all creatures of habit. We all prefer certain *sleep cues* or *sleep associations,* and so do our babies.

The 2004 Sleep in America poll of 1,500 families to find the most common sleep cues parents used with their babies. They found:

- Sixty percent of parents rock their infants to sleep.
- Seventy-five percent of infants fall asleep nursing or drinking a bottle.
- Fifteen to thirty percent of parents bed share most nights.

Parents often worry that putting their baby to bed with rocking, nursing, and the like creates "bad" habits. Some doctors warn that lulling a baby to sleep will become a crutch and undermine his ability to self-soothe at a two A.M. waking. But there's a huge difference between *good* sleep cues and *bad* sleep crutches. Good cues help babies fall asleep fast—and slumber longer—yet are easy to use and easy to wean. Bad sleep cues, on the other hand, are inconvenient, exhausting, and hard to wean. For example, if your baby can only fall asleep with thirty minutes of bottom patting and needs it several times a night, I think it's pretty clear you're looking at a bad sleep cue.

Research confirms that *certain* sleep associations do create sleep problems. A British study found that babies who were rocked and nursed to sleep each night had more sleep problems at three months of age. A large Norwegian study found that babies who bed share at six months had *triple* the risk of night waking at eighteen months.

Fortunately the 5 S's are the best of all sleep cues. They're easy to use, easy to wean, and work fast. Here's how to use them to boost your baby's sleep:

1st *S:* Swaddling

The world is just too big for little babies. In the womb, your baby always slept snugly cuddled. The soft walls of the womb held her arms and legs, preventing startles and twitches. No wonder being unwrapped in a big crib feels so bizarre and "free-floating."

Studies show the womb-like embrace of wrapping boosts sleep. One German review found swaddling reduced nighttime waking by 50 percent, and other studies have reported it boosts sleep by up to forty-five minutes.

But, contrary to expectations, swaddled babies sleep better . . . *but not more deeply.* In other words, wrapped babies are not so deep in sleep that they "forget to breathe." In fact, one study found swaddling boosted sleep *and* boosted a baby's awareness of his environment.

Exhausted moms place babies on their stomachs or fall asleep with them on a bed or sofa when they fuss a lot. By reducing crying and boosting sleep, swaddling reduces an exhausted mom's temptation to place her sleeping baby on the stomach or fall asleep with him on the sofa or in their bed. A Washington, D.C., study found that moms who swaddle are significantly more likely to keep babies safely on their backs!

Lastly, swaddling lessens a baby's ability to roll to the stomach. (Nighttime rolling raises a baby's SIDS risk eight to forty-five times!) If your baby *can* roll while wrapped, you need to make sure you're swaddling correctly and playing rough, rumbly white noise. However, if the rolling continues, ask your doctor about letting your baby sleep in a *fully reclined* swing or a smart sleeper.

Note: Swaddling must always be done safely: Don't overheat your baby, avoid bulky blankets, and make sure her hips and legs can easily flex and open.

2nd *S*: Side/Stomach Position

The side and stomach are the best positions for soothing a baby, but the back is the *only* safe position for naps and nights. The AAP says it's safe to sleep tummy down once your baby can roll over, but I strongly disagree. Athletic babies can roll as early as two or three months—the peak age of SIDS! Fortunately, swaddling and white noise help reduce a baby's fidgetiness and ability to roll over until four or five months, when 80 to 90 percent of SIDS risk has passed.

Note: Do supervised tummy time every day to help your baby strengthen her neck and back muscles. That will help her develop the lifesaving ability to lift her head off the mattress and move her face to the side.

3rd *S*: Shushing

Some parents think swaddling is all their baby needs. *But that's a big mistake!*

During the first months, white noise is as important as swaddling. And, from four to twelve months of age, sound is the most important sleep cue! That's because babies—who sleep great with just wrapping—can suddenly fall apart when the swaddling is stopped at four months. They start *popping awake* from any little outside distraction (noisy neighbors, passing planes, hallway lights) or internal discomforts (teething, mild colds, a touch of hunger, or a little gas). And once aroused, your four-month-old may replace the silence of her room with wails begging you to come in for a cuddle . . . and to play.

Luckily, white noise distracts babies from all these disturbances. And, if your baby does awaken, the familiar rumble will help her return to sleep.

Sound helps sleep by:

• Keeping the calming reflex turned on (during the early months of life).
• Reducing wiggling that can cause accidental rolling.
• Keeping babies sleeping well long after the wrapping is stopped. (Once swaddling is weaned, white noise becomes *the* key sleep cue . . . like a teddy bear of sound.)

Surprisingly, the Sleep in America poll showed that less than a third of parents used this independence-building sleep cue.

Babies sleep best with rumbly sounds. "Nature" sounds, such as ocean waves or cricket chirps, are often ineffective. (Note: Music can lull babies to sleep, but when used all night, the changing tones can actually wake your baby up.)

To be most effective, play sound all night . . . for all sleep . . . the entire first year (or longer). Little sheep that shut off after thirty minutes may accidentally reduce sleep if a baby rouses in the middle of the night and is "suddenly" upset by the unaccustomed silence. White noise machines are also problematic if they are too hissy and high pitched. As noted in chapter 10, high-pitched sound is great for calming crying, but to promote sleep, you need sound that mimics the deep rumble of the womb (around 65 dB).

Of course, you shouldn't blast loud noise all night. To avoid the risk of excessive sound use a smart sleeper that automatically increases and decreases the sound, tailoring it to your baby's changing levels of fussiness, throughout the night.

Note: As with swaddling, only use white noise during fussy periods and sleep, not 24/7. It's also a good idea to play white noise—quietly in the background—during the bedtime routine. It signals to your baby that his sweet glide into dreamland is about to begin.

Preventing Depression: A Surprising Benefit of White Noise

Exhaustion and depression can create a terrible vicious cycle for new mothers. We all get more depressed when we're weary, but postpartum depression is especially disturbing because worrisome thoughts often visit in the night and shatter your sleep . . . leading to an ever worsening cycle of fatigue and anxiety.

Health educators at New Jersey's Virtua Health reported that depressed moms who were taught the *5 S's* had less anxiety and marital stress, more sleep and confidence, and fewer urges to harm their babies. Virtua's nurses noted that, besides helping the babies, rumbly white noise helped quiet the anxious thoughts that disturbed moms in the dark hours of the night . . . and gave them the sleep they needed to get on the road to recovery.

One dad wrote, "Sound was the secret sauce for getting our little Selene to sleep. And what was really cool was that the rain sound that soothed our baby also snookered my depressed, insomniac wife. She started falling asleep much faster and stopped waking up with every passing train."

Do You Hate Noise at Night?

Some adults are sound sensitive. The slightest floor board creaks or drumming of someone's fingers on a table can be very annoying. They often say that *total silence* is their favorite sleep cue, and they're hesitant to play white noise when their new baby is sleeping right next to their bed.

But these adults are not so much *noise* sensitive as they are *high-pitch* sensitive. They fall asleep in trains and planes and love the sound of the rain . . . but hissing sounds drive them crazy.

If high-pitch noises get on *your* nerves, here are some steps to help you make friends with your baby's white noise:

- Pick the right sound. Use a low-pitch sound (my favorite is rain on the roof that is specially engineered to be extra deep and rumbly.
- Play it softly each evening. A few hours of background white noise (even during TV) will help your brain to get used to it.
- Start using it all night. After a week of background white noise, start using it softly all night, gradually increasing the volume to the level of a shower sound over another week's time. (If you still find the sound annoying, put a towel over your speakers to filter out more of the high-pitched tones.)
- Try earplugs: If all else fails, use a pair of good earplugs to screen out the sound. (Just makes sure someone can hear your baby when she cries.)

4th *S*: Swinging

Swinging is super-effective for calming crying. In fact, for some "bouncy baby boys" it's the only thing that soothes screaming. The same is true with sleeping. *All* babies love being rocked to sleep, but 10 to 20 percent don't just love it . . . they need it! Unfortunately, vibration and gentle swinging are too subtle to help these babies very much. Even swaddling and sound fail to help these kids, unless they're also jiggled.

If your baby is a poor sleeper, despite sound and swaddling, use a smart sleeper that delivers safe swaddling, optimized white noise, and soothing rocking all night long. Or ask your doctor's permission for your baby to sleep in a *fully reclined* infant swing. (Of course, you must buckle her in securely.) Note: The AAP warns parents *not* to use car seats, infant seats, or swings as sleeping locations for long naps or nights.

5th *S*: Sucking

Sucking on a breast or a bottle of milk is profoundly calming. And infants who go to bed sucking on a pacifier have a lower risk of SIDS . . . even if it drops out of their mouth soon after sleep begins!

Believe it or not, your baby's teeth may start coming in as early as three or four months. That's when you have to start preventing cavities. Once your infant's teeth come through, keep the sucking periods to under thirty minutes at a time. Sucking on a bottle or breast for long periods bathes the soft new teeth in sugar solution and encourages cavity-causing bacteria to grow. If your little one wants more sucking, offer a pacifier or a bottle of water or unsweetened herbal tea, like mint or chamomile, made with boiled water, then cooled, during the first three months of life.

The *5 S's* for Safer Sleep

Dutch and American studies have reported some pretty bad news: Parents often put fussy babies to bed in the riskier stomach position. But the good news is that if we can reduce baby crying and improve baby sleep, we may be able to reduce a mom's temptation to use unsafe sleeping habits. In fact, that is exactly what was reported in a study in Washington, D.C. Moms who swaddled their babies were significantly more likely to use the safer back-sleeping position.

Fortunately, by improving infant sleep we can encourage exhausted parents to follow our life-saving "back to sleep" advice.

WEANING SLEEPING BABIES OFF THE 5 S'S

Once the fourth trimester is over, the calming reflex gradually changes from an automatic response to a familiar, reassuring sleep cue that works only when your infant is ready to be soothed. (Shushing is magical with a fussy two-month-old, but doing it to an angry ten-month-old will just make you both more upset!)

Increasingly, your bedtime routine becomes the key to good sleep as your smart infant gets better and better at remembering patterns. *Ahh, my bath, that lullaby, the shushing . . . I feel tired already.*

But just as kids outgrow training wheels on their bikes, they must eventually learn to sleep with fewer sleep cues. The first S you'll wean is swinging. If your doctor gave you permission to use a *fully reclined* swing, three or four months is usually the time to start weaning from it. Just reduce the speed to the slowest setting for a few days. If your baby continues to sleep well, let him sleep in the nonmoving swing. A few days later, if he's still sleeping soundly, move him to the bassinet or crib. (Your smart sleeper automatically weans motion after four months.)

Most infants are ready to say good-bye to swaddling by four or five months. Until then, wrapping is useful because it calms crying, boosts sleep, *and* reduces the risk of accidental rolling. (Eighty percent of infant sleep deaths occur during the first four months.)

Wean swaddling in two steps: First, do the snug wrap . . . with one arm out. Then, if all goes well for a few days, you can stop it completely. If one arm wrapping makes your baby wake more, try full swaddling for another month.

Note: It's *much* easier to wean swaddling when you play rumbly white noise for naps and nights. Once out of the wrap, your social four-month-old will probably wake up much more in a stone silent room.

Sucking is the next *S* to phase out, usually by six months. Bedtime pacifier use lowers SIDS risk (even if the paci is dropped soon after sleep begins). And by six months your baby will be past 90 percent of the risk of SIDS. Sometimes, waiting more than six or seven months makes weaning the paci a lot harder because it allows more of an emotional attachment to develop.

The last *S* you'll wean is shushing. Rough white noise boosts sleep, even through teething, growth spurts, and mild colds. So I don't stop sound until twelve months . . . or later.

Sound is super-easy to wean. Just dial down the volume—little by little—over one to two weeks, and soon the noise will be history. If you ever want to restart it—on a trip or during an illness—just gradually crank it back up over a few days.

Note: A white noise CD helps toddlers—even older kids—sleep well on vacations or in stressful situations (like a new sibling, illness, noisy neighbors, or fears).

THE TRUTH ABOUT PUTTING YOUR BABY ON SCHEDULES

Toddlers love routines, but what about babies? Should schedules be shunned or embraced? Like so many child-rearing issues, there's more than one right answer.

Scheduling is a modern concept. The ancients didn't feed babies according to the time on the sundial. But staying organized can be a lifesaver for today's moms and help a baby adopt a schedule that works better for the family.

Of course, *rigid* schedules that ignore a baby's cries are unnatural and unloving. But *flexible* schedules—that set approximate times for feeding and sleep—can work quite well.

A study of breast-fed babies found that two simple scheduling tweaks yielded a big improvement in sleep in the first two months:

- Waking for a "dream feed," between ten P.M. and midnight.
- Responding to nighttime cries with a few minutes of holding or a diaper change *before* feeding.

Within three weeks, 100 percent of babies were sleeping five-hour stretches with these two steps, versus just 23 percent of infants where no scheduling was tried.

When you think about it, the benefit of flexible schedules isn't a huge surprise since babies are learning experts! Even before birth, your baby starts recognizing your voice and favorite music. So learning the pattern of feeding and sleeping is not above her pay grade.

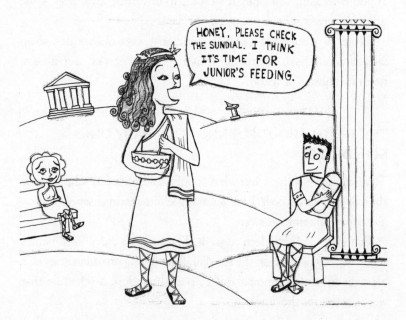

Some experts advise an "eat, play, sleep" schedule. They hope that by using a little play to separate eating from sleeping (rather than always feeding before sleep) will help babies learn to fall sleep—without a feeding—when they wake at two A.M..

This sounds logical, but it actually goes against your baby's biology. Infants get sleepy after feedings, no matter how much you prod and play with them. Also, before bedtime, you will want to fill your little guy's tummy to prolong his sleep.

If you are going to try scheduling, I suggest you wait about a month (until feeding is going really well), then do the following:

- Carry your baby a lot during the day to help him learn the difference between day and night.
- During the day, feed your love bug every one and a half to two hours, then put him to sleep. (Start the nap *before* he's yawning and looking droopy eyed.)
- If he naps over two hours, wake him for his next play/feed period. Long naps cause less daytime eating and more hunger at night.
- Feed him in a quiet room so he doesn't get distracted and refuse to eat.
- Turn the white noise on—and the lights down—twenty minutes before naps and bedtime. This quiets your baby's nervous system and gives a clear signal that sleepy-time is coming. Use the wake-and-sleep technique (see page 212) to help him learn to self-soothe.
- Wake your baby for a "dream feed" between ten P.M. and midnight every night to fill his stomach and prepare him for a longer sleep period.

A flexible eating and sleeping schedule can be super-helpful if you have twins, other kids, you're a single parent, or you're working out of the house. But, the key word is *flexible*. If you're planning a one P.M. nap, but your little guy is exhausted at twelve thirty, it's fine to bend the "rules." Just feed him and put him down early. And if he get's hungry before his "scheduled" feeding time, try distracting him, but respond with promptness and love if the fussing persists, and return to the schedule later.

Note: Rigid schedules (you never deviate even if your baby is crying with hunger) are contrary to our natural instincts, make us constantly watch the clock, and lead to underfed babies.

To establish a schedule, follow the same reassuring routine every night:

Low lights

Soft white noise in the background

Toasty bath

Loving massage with warm oil

Yummy milk

Cozy swaddle

A soft lullaby

Within a week, these will begin to work like hypnosis. As you start the routine your baby will think, *Wow, I'm sleepy already!*

SIDS AND SUFFOCATION: A PARENT'S NIGHTMARE

For about seventy years, the mysterious condition called SIDS (sudden infant death syndrome) has been the leading cause of death in babies one to twelve months of age. SIDS peaks between two and four months, with 90 percent of deaths occurring before six months of age.

During the 1980s, five thousand U.S. babies died from SIDS

every year. Back then, we warned moms to never let babies sleep *on the back*. We thought they might choke on spitup and die. (Besides, every grandma knew that babies slept better on their stomach.)

Then in the 1990s, doctors realized *we had been tragically wrong*. Back-sleeping babies don't choke if they spit up during sleep. They just swallow it or let it dribble out. On the contrary, we discovered that *stomach* sleeping was the big problem. In fact, stomach sleeping raises the risk of SIDS three to eight times!

Doctors did an immediate about-face and began imploring parents to *only* let babies sleep on the back. Within a few years, the Back to Sleep initiative was one of the greatest successes in medical history: SIDS deaths dropped 50 percent . . . saving the lives of thousands of babies a year!

Unfortunately, over the past twenty years, that great progress has plateaued. SIDS deaths have barely dropped further and suffocation deaths (from sofa sleeping and bed sharing) have quadrupled. The government says two thousand babies still die of SIDS every year, but now about fifteen hundred additional infants die during sleep of suffocation or unknown causes.

The 9/11 tragedy led to three thousand deaths. That is exactly the number of innocent babies who die during sleep . . . every single year! And the situation is getting worse, as more parents bed share or choose risky sleep spots including sofas, recliners, bean bags, air mattresses, water beds, car seats, infant carriers, and poorly designed slings. Scottish researchers found a higher risk of SIDS—sixty-seven times higher!—among babies who were allowed to sleep on a couch. And this has been confirmed in American studies.

Note: Be careful! About half of all moms who nurse their babies on a couch or arm chair fall asleep there . . . and the consequences can be dire.

A Dozen Ways to Stop SIDS and Suffocation

SIDS is not a topic anyone wants to think about—but thankfully there are many ways to dramatically reduce your baby's risk:

1. Only let your baby sleep on the back.
2. Breast-feed if you can: This reduces SIDS by 50 percent.
3. Have a smoke-free house: Don't smoke or allow others to do so. Avoid woodstoves, incense, candles, and fireplaces, unless the room is well vented.
4. Avoid overheating or overcooling: Keep the room 68°F to 72°F (20°C to 22.2°C) and avoid hats and overdressing. Your baby's ears should feel slightly warm (not cold or hot).
5. Sleep in the same room as your baby for at least the first six months.
6. Use snug swaddling for nighttime and naps.
7. Offer a pacifier at bedtime. If you're breast-feeding, wait a couple of weeks until the nursing is well established before giving a paci.
8. Don't sleep with your baby for the first nine months. Never let him sleep on a couch, recliner, sofa, armchair, beanbag chair, or water bed.
9. Remove pillows, toys, stuffed animals, bumpers, and thick or loose bedding that could cause smothering, such as duvets, pillows, positioners, and lambskins from your baby's sleeping area. And never place thick blankets *under* the baby.
10. Practice supervised tummy time to help your baby develop the muscle strength to be able to move his face away from choking risks.
11. Don't let your baby sleep sitting up in a car seat, infant carrier, or swing, especially if she's a preemie or developmentally delayed.
12. Use a smart sleeper equipped with a special sleep sack that prevents accidental rolling over.

Unfortunately, there's no guaranteed way to prevent SIDS. But most victims have two or more of the risk factors listed above, so following these tips can definitely make your baby safer!

Five More Sleep Safety Tips

Here are five more ways to keep your sleeping baby safe:

- Never leave her alone on an adult bed. (Even during the first months, babies can accidentally wiggle or roll over and fall.)
- Use smoke alarms and periodically check that they're working.
- Install a carbon monoxide detector in the hall near your bedroom.
- Store an easy-to-grab fire extinguisher on each floor.
- Make an emergency plan (for earthquakes, tornadoes, hurricanes, and fires). If you live high above the ground, keep a rope ladder and a fire evacuation hood on hand.

Note: Being safe gives you peace of mind . . . and a little money back, too! Many insurance companies offer refunds when you purchase smoke alarms and fire extinguishers.

ROOM SHARING: "I JUST GOT EVICTED—CAN I SLEEP AT YOUR PLACE?"

Thou shalt sleep with thy fathers.

Deuteronomy 31:16

Should your baby sleep in your room or her nursery?

Since mankind's earliest days, parents and babies have slept together for mutual protection, warmth, and convenience. However, at the start of the twentieth century, U.S. parents were told that children should sleep in their own rooms to keep them from becoming spoiled. So parents ended thousands of years of closeness and moved their babies to cribs in their own rooms. Today, some American parents still think sleep's a time for children to learn about privacy and self-reliance. (And some even view sharing the bedroom as a parental sacrifice!)

But after nine long months of pregnancy it's too abrupt a change to deposit your baby in another room. Also, sharing a bedroom is more convenient for two A.M. diapering and feeding (you don't have to toddle down a cold hallway). *Plus* . . . room sharing is safer! During the first six months, having your baby next to your bed reduces the risk of SIDS.

Don't worry about your baby getting used to being in your room. You'll have little trouble transitioning her to her own room if you start using her nursery for naps at around five months and for nights around six months. Ending room sharing after that can still be done, but the longer you wait the tougher it may become for your baby to make the switch. (Switching will be easier if you continue the same white noise you've been using in your bedroom.)

Most moms find they sleep better knowing their baby is right next to them. And the white noise can even help tired parents fall back asleep after middle-of-the-night feedings.

BED SHARING—GREAT IDEA OR RISKY BUSINESS?

As I just mentioned, bed sharing is one of the oldest of parenting practices. A century ago, the custom was almost abandoned in the West, but recently its popularity has grown dramatically; doubling over the past twenty years. The graphs on page 233 and 235 show that, in 2010, 25 percent of families with infants under the age of six months routinely brought the baby into their bed (33 percent Hispanics, 38 percent blacks, 17 percent whites).

Why has bed sharing doubled? Some moms do it to make nursing easier, and others because it seems "more natural." But most

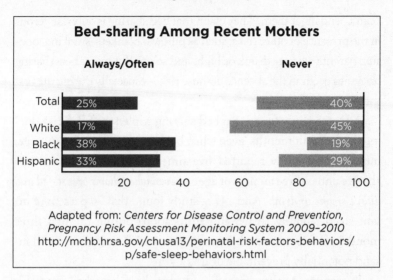

Bed-sharing Among Recent Mothers

Always/Often | Never

Total 25% — 40%
White 17% — 45%
Black 38% — 19%
Hispanic 33% — 29%

20 40 60 80 100

Adapted from: *Centers for Disease Control and Prevention, Pregnancy Risk Assessment Monitoring System 2009–2010*
http://mchb.hrsa.gov/chusa13/perinatal-risk-factors-behaviors/
p/safe-sleep-behaviors.html

bed share because they're desperate to get more sleep! Yet the nation's top doctors warn that up to 70 percent of all sleep deaths happen when babies are brought into an adult bed.

So, what's right? Is bed sharing a wonderful ancient tradition and a true bonding experience? Or is it a risk that can lead to tragedy?

Personally, I worry about bed sharing for two reasons. First, it leads to more sleeping problems. As mentioned earlier, researchers have found more night waking at three months of age among bed sharers. And in a large study of U.S. and Norwegian families, bed sharing at six months tripled the chances of night waking issues at eighteen months. A Penn State study found a higher rate of dissatisfaction and postpartum depression among bed sharing moms. And a New Zealand study uncovered a different type of sleep problem. Although bed sharing is called "the family bed," researchers found that in a quarter of bed sharing families, dads move out of the bed into another room! (So much for the *family* bed.)

Second, and much more concerning, is the increased risk of death that comes with bed sharing. Some experts pooh-pooh this risk, saying that these moms are "aware" of their babies all night and therefore "can't" endanger them. They claim that bed sharing is only dangerous in the presence of other risks, such as pillows/blankets, smoking, obesity, parents who are drunk or high, and so on. But many bed-sharing tragedies occur in the absence of those risk—especially during the first three months.

A Dutch study found that bed sharing tripled the SIDS risk during the first four months, even when babies were breast-fed. A large, multinational study reported five times more SIDS risk for bed sharers under three months of age . . . *even when moms breast-fed and didn't smoke or drink.* And a U.S. study found that 70 percent of infant sleep fatalities (SIDS and suffocation) during the first three months of life occurred while sharing the bed. That's over two thousand potentially preventable deaths a year!

In response to these tragedies, doctors have launched a massive campaign to teach parents about safe sleep. The hope has been that teaching parents about sleep safety (the "ABC" advice: *A*lone, *B*ack sleeping, in a *C*rib) would lead to fewer deaths.

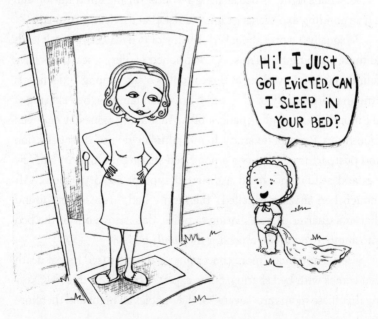

But public education overlooks an absolutely critical point: Parents are ignoring doctors' bed-sharing concerns because . . . we're ignoring their concerns! While we chant our Back to Sleep mantra, parents counter with "Hey! My baby hates sleeping on her back, unswaddled, in an empty crib, in a quiet room. She only sleeps well in bed with me. And I need her to sleep because I'm exhausted!"

Bottom line: Weary parents ignore medical advice because they're sleep deprived. They're not bad parents, they're just desperate to soothe their babies and get enough rest to function the next day. And these moms and dads feel abandoned by doctors who advise them to "let the baby cry to sleep" and "just wait a few months" for colicky screaming to go away.

Fortunately, with the 5 *S*'s we have the ability to keep babies safe *and* to help parents get the sleep they need. Doctors simply must add suggestions on improving baby sleep to our safe sleep message. By boosting sleep (with swaddling, white noise, and motion) we can remove a parent's temptation to take unnecessary chances.

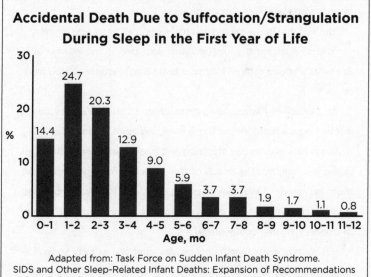

Accidental Death Due to Suffocation/Strangulation During Sleep in the First Year of Life

Adapted from: Task Force on Sudden Infant Death Syndrome. SIDS and Other Sleep-Related Infant Deaths: Expansion of Recommendations for a Safe Infant Sleeping Environment. *Pediatrics*, 2011; 128: e1341–e1367.

Note: For older infants, the family bed can be both beautiful and safe. As the graph on page 235 shows, most accidental suffocation and strangulation in bed (ASSB) occurs under six months, and rarely up to twelve months of age. So if you're thinking of bed sharing, I encourage you to wait at least nine months. (The AAP recommends delaying until the first birthday.)

Drunk Parenting: Another Bed-Sharing Risk

Every sitcom in history has joked about exhausted new parents brushing their teeth with a tube of sunscreen or the like. One new mom I know was so tired that, when pulling into a parking space, she blacked out for a few seconds and drove her car right into the building! And then there's the famous T-shirt of a distraught mom saying "Oh no! I left my baby on the bus!"

Half of all new moms sleep less than six hours a night for weeks in a row—sometimes for months. And that may be on top of months of poor sleep at the end of pregnancy.

But did you know exhaustion makes you as ditzy as a drunk?

You'd never bring your baby into your bed if you were drunk. But what if you're so tired that your brain is as wasted *as if* you were drunk?

University of Pennsylvania researchers evaluated adults sleeping six hours a night versus those snoozing eight hours. When they tested their ability to pay attention and think clearly, the well-rested group did fine, but the brains of the six-hour group got more and more impaired . . . with every passing day. After two weeks of sleep deprivation, the attention of the six-hour group *dropped to the level of people who are legally drunk*!

Of course, the research only proves what you already know: Exhaustion makes us stagger, stutter, and slur our words, and undermines our judgment, reaction time, and memory. Alarmingly, the

2004 Sleep in America poll found that 48 percent of parents admit to driving while drowsy and 10 percent confessed to falling asleep at the wheel!

So, does fatigue put your baby at risk if you're bed sharing? Unfortunately it can.

New Zealand researchers placed video cameras in the bedrooms of bed-sharing families. For two-thirds of the night (almost six hours) the moms kept their babies in the riskier side-lying position. (One in forty babies actually rolled all the way to their stomachs.) Nighttime videotaping by British doctors discovered that a third of bed-sharing moms accidentally rested an arm or leg on their baby during sleep. And most bed-sharing babies had their faces covered with bedding at some time during the night. (In each case, this was caused by the parent.) New Zealand researchers confirmed this finding, noting that the faces of the bed-sharing babies were covered for nearly one hour per night.

You might say, "Hmmm . . . I know I'm tired, but I don't feel *that tired*." But here's the kicker: People who are drunk tired are terrible at estimating how weary they really are. When we're exhausted, parts of your brain can fall into sleep, even while you're still awake (this is called microsleep). That makes you underestimate how much your mental sharpness has dulled.

Note: To keep from falling asleep in bed with their baby, some moms toddle out to the living room to do the middle-of-the-night feeding on a sofa or recliner. *But even there you need to keep alert!* Almost half of all mothers nursing on a sofa fall asleep during the feeding. And babies sleeping on sofas or chairs have a very elevated risk of SIDS.

LOWER THE RISK: IF YOU'RE DETERMINED TO BED SHARE

Bed sharing advocates often point to studies that find it as safe as cribs. They note that Japanese parents frequently bed share, yet have low rates of SIDS—although that may be because they use firm futons. They also note that bed sharing is safer than sofa sharing— although they admit both are associated with increased deaths. A couple of SIDS studies found no increased risk with bed sharing, as long as parents are sober, attentive, and nonsmoking, although exhaustion was not evaluated in these studies.

If you're strongly drawn to bed sharing despite these concerns, here are some tips to help you decrease the risks:

- Breast-feed—it can reduce SIDS by 50 percent.
- Don't smoke or use alcohol or drugs . . . not even antihistamines.
- Remove bulky bedding such as pillows and blankets.
- Avoid water beds, bean bags, air mattresses, couches, or recliners.
- Never leave your baby unattended in your bed.
- Make sure your baby can't fall (a risk as early as one or two months).
- Prevent accidental wedging between the bed and a wall or headboard.
- Get rest! Exhaustion makes you as risky as someone who is drunk.
- Use a bedtime pacifier.
- Never bed share with a preemie or a low-birth-weight newborn
- Keep the room at 68°F to 72°F (19°C to 22.2°C). Touch your baby's ears and nose to make sure they're neither cold nor hot.

- No bed sharing with a sibling, animal, or anyone who is obese.
- Keep your baby on the side of one parent, not in between both.
- Make sure the immunizations of your baby—and all family and caregivers—are up-to-date.
- Don't use candles, incense, or a wood-burning fire.
- Swaddle to prevent accidental rolling.
- Avoid choking risks, such as clothing that might cover your baby's face or tangle around her neck, or cords from drapery/blinds.

Twins: Double Your Pleasure . . . If You Can Get Some Sleep

The U.S. government reports that one in thirty births are twins—the highest rate on record! As you might imagine, multiples make it extra tough to get enough sleep. (Or even to pee!) Researchers from Case Western Reserve found that moms of twins slept only 6.2 hours a night during the first months. And it was even worse for their husbands, who clocked in a measly 5.8 hours in an entire day.

If you have twins—or more—here's how to boost your babies' sleep . . . and yours:

1. Use swaddling and white noise for all sleeping and fussy periods.
2. Put your babies on a flexible schedule. (More about this on page 225.)
3. Use the *wake-and-sleep* technique to help your babies learn to self-soothe. (See page 212.)
4. After you feed one baby, wake the other to eat, too.
5. Nap when you can!

6. Ask for help! Family, friends, and babysitters can give you little breaks ... so you don't break.

7. Get your babies—and all caregivers and family members—immunized.

8. Use a smart sleeper.

Note: If you have the babies sleep in the same crib, make sure they're properly swaddled ... and don't do it past the first month. A British study videotaping sixty pairs of sleeping twins from newborn to five months found that twins sleeping side by side occasionally covered each other's face with a free arm! This caused mild breathing problems (lowered oxygen) and required the affected twin to awaken and turn her head or push her sibling's arm away. (Obviously they weren't swaddled.)

Preemies: Getting Your Little Baby's Sleep in Gear

Preemies look so tiny and vulnerable—no wonder parents feel intimidated (especially if the baby is sick and had to stay in the newborn ICU).

And life gets even more exhausting after the baby leaves the hospital. During their first weeks at home, preemies often wake every two to three hours—all night long. Babies get so accustomed to the light and activity in the NICU that the dark stillness of the home can actually be disturbing. Another problem that often emerges after coming home is a spike in fussiness. Crying typically accelerates around the time preemies are discharged from the hospital. That's not because the nurses were so gifted (although many of them are); it's because preemies enter the normal fussy period around their due date, which is about when they go home.

Fortunately, some tips can help you survive the early months:

• During the day, do lots of nursing, holding, rocking, and skin-to-skin contact to keep the calming reflex turned on.

- Reduce overstimulation from the commotion of your home.
- Use swaddling and white noise for all naps and night sleeping, as well as for fussy periods.
- Nap when you can.
- Get help when you can.
- Make sure the immunizations of your baby—and all caregivers and family members—are up-to-date.
- Keep germs and illness out of your house by reducing visitors (especially children) and insisting that everyone wash hands.
- Have a smoke-free home (no cigarettes, pot, candles, wood-burning fires).
- Promote better sleeping with a smart sleeper.

The Whys About the S's: Questions Parents Ask About Sleep

1. *When I put my sleeping baby down, he's often up and yelling within minutes. Why?*

   Even sleeping babies have some awareness of their surroundings. Your baby clearly feels the difference between your warm, embracing sway and the quiet, flat bassinet. You can help avoid this problem by swaddling, using a pacifier, and turning on rumbly white noise *before* you place him into the bassinet. Those all reduce the abrupt change your baby experiences when you transfer him into the bassinet. Also, use the *wake-and-sleep* technique to boost his ability to self-soothe. (See page 212.) Or, use a smart sleeper to ease his transition to sleep.

2. *When my baby falls asleep at the end of a feeding, should I do a burping and risk waking him up?*

   Yes, burp him to keep him from spitting up in his sleep. While you're at it, also check to see if he needs a diaper change. Don't worry about waking your baby. After a feeding, he will feel a little "drunk," and he should slide back into sleep quickly when you use the 5 S's and *wake-and-sleep.*

Note: It's also a good idea to put ointment on your baby's bottom at bedtime, to protect his skin from any middle-of-the-night pee or poop.

3. *I worry about overbundling my baby in the warm weather. How can I tell if he's overheated?*

It's actually quite easy: Feel his little ears. If they are red or very warm, he's too hot; if they're cold, he's too chilly; and if they feel "fresh" (neither hot, nor cold), his body temperature is just right.

Even on warm days, your baby will benefit from swaddling. So, dress him in just a diaper, wrap him in a light cotton blanket (or one with cooling netting), and check his ears to make sure he's not too hot.

4. *Does sleep get disturbed when babies have a growth spurt?*

Newborns grow super-fast, doubling their weight in six months or less. Some babies grow at an even, steady pace, but many grow in monthly fits and starts (growth spurts and plateaus). In the midst of such a growth spurt, you can expect your baby to wake more frequently and cry for more milk. (That's really a *demand* feeding!)

5. *Why does my baby get up at the crack of dawn?*

Even when babies are asleep they still feel, hear—and see! The early morning light filters through their closed eyes and thin skull and acts like an alarm clock. Fortunately, sound and swaddling (and the calming motions of a smart sleeper) can coax many early risers back into sleep. (Rumbly white noise also obscures early morning sounds of birds, dogs, traffic, and neighbors.) Also, try blackout curtains.

However, if you can't charm your infant back to sleep,

you may need to bid adieu to your warm bed and take your little "rooster baby" out for an early-morning constitutional.

6. *Is it wrong for my baby to sleep in his infant carrier?*

Walking with your baby in a sling is a great way to give a big helping of fourth trimester jiggly motion, cuddling, and rhythmic sound. That's why it's almost impossible to keep babies awake when they're toted around.

Don't worry about accidentally teaching bad habits. After the fourth trimester ends, your four-month-old will have many additional skills to entertain himself, without needing to be carried.

Note: Babies can suffocate inside slings if they sink in too far and their heads get bent forward. Make sure you can always see your child's face so you can check for any breathing problem.

7. *Is it okay to let my baby sleep on my chest?*

Sleeping with your baby on your chest is so sweet, but it does lead to unwanted risks. Stomach-lying babies have a higher risk of suffocation and SIDS. I also worry about babies falling off their parent's chest. I once got a call in the middle of the night when a four-week-old fell off his sleeping father's chest and hit the wall next to the bed. Luckily, the baby wasn't hurt, but—as you can imagine—the parents felt terrible.

8. *Should I stop swaddling once my baby can roll over?*

No baby should sleep on the stomach during the first four to six months (unless your doctor specifically advises it for medical reasons). Babies begin to roll to the risky stomach position at two to four months of age. Swaddling makes it hard for them to flip their legs over to get the motion started, often delaying rolling to prone by an extra month or two. But what if your two-month-old acrobat can roll even when swaddled? In that case, I recommend three things: a) Make sure you are swaddling correctly—snug swaddling with the arms straight down at the side makes flipping much harder, b) use white noise—this makes babies less fidgety . . . and less likely to roll, and c) use a smart sleeper—the sleeper's secure sleep sack keeps babies safer by preventing rolling to the stomach.

9. *My seven-week-old catnaps for thirty minutes and wakes up cranky and tired. How can I get her to nap longer?*

Catnapping is common and it may occur because the room is too stimulating . . . or too quiet! By two to three months, babies become more social, and TV—or toddler—noise can snap her out of a nap. On the other hand, some babies can't nap if the house is too quiet! Hopefully, adding rumbly white noise will improve your daughter's napping by keeping her calming reflex on.

A PARENT'S PERSPECTIVE: MEMOIRS FROM THE MATTRESS

> *We went through fire and water almost in trying to procure for him a natural sleep. We swung him in blankets, wheeled him in little carts, walked the room with him by the hour, etc., etc., but it was wonderful how little sleep he obtained after all. He always looked wide awake and as if he did not need sleep.*
>
> G. L. Prentiss, *The Life and Letters of Elizabeth Prentiss*, 1822

Poor Elizabeth Prentiss could have learned a thing or two from these parents who transformed their babies' nighttime sleep:

"As she reached the four-week mark, our daughter, Eve, became more wakeful and distressed. When she wasn't eating or sleeping, she was fussing—or screaming. One night, she yelled so much her nose got stuffed and she started to snort. I cradled her in my arms—resting them on top of a moving clothing dryer—and called the doctor. The noise, vibration, and warmth of the dryer calmed her enough to allow me to talk to the nurse.

"She told me about how to use the 5 S's, without using the dryer. Over the next couple of weeks, I became skilled at doing them, and Eve rewarded us with six- to seven-hour stretches of nighttime sleep."

Shari and Michael, parents of Hillary, Noah, and Eve

When Wyatt was two months old, his parents—Lise, a nurse, and Aaron, a physician—noticed he would sleep five hours at night when wrapped and serenaded by white noise but only three hours when his arms were free and the room was quiet.

Lise said, "I was happy with how well he was doing, but I also worried he would get addicted to the sensations and have trouble sleeping without them when he got older. So when he turned three months, I stopped it all.

"Everything seemed fine, until Wyatt turned four months. Out of the blue, he began waking—and screaming—every two hours, all night long! One friend told me he was teething, but acetaminophen didn't help. My husband guessed he was going through a growth spurt, but rice cereal didn't help, either. At Wyatt's four-month checkup, the doctor suggested we stop the medicine and cereal and try the wrapping and white noise again.

"To be honest, I thought Wyatt was too old for swaddling, but I was desperate. Within two nights, our little boy went from crying five times a night to waking just once, chowing down his milk, and then immediately sacking out again until six A.M.! He loved the rain sound on the CD. It helped me to sleep, too!"

Lise and Aaron, parents of Wyatt and Rachel

~~~~~~~~~~

The Fourth Trimester Ends . . .
and a Rainbow Appears

He's starting to love us back a little.

Francie, mother of four-month-old Jackson

HOORAY! YOUR BABY IS READY TO BE BORN!

At birth, Esmé was a pudgy, sweet-smelling baby who needed to use all her concentration to gaze into her mother's eyes. By four months, she could shoot broad grins out at anyone in the room, as if to say, "Ain't I great!"

It has been four long months since you cut the umbilical cord, but finally your baby is really ready to be born. He has brilliantly adapted to the huge change from your womb to the world.

At last, there is a light at the end of the long tunnel that was the fourth trimester, and, happily, that light is . . . a beautiful rainbow. What your baby has achieved in his brief lifetime is truly amazing! He started out as helpless as a mouse, and now his brain has grown

25 percent in size and he is a happy, responsive member of the family.

Increasingly, your baby's relaxed, open hands allow him to latch on to his rattle (or your nose), and he now uses his adorable, toothless grin to make everyone fall in love with him! After months of fuzzy stares and long sleeps, your four-month-old's laugh and gurgle announce to the world, "Dress rehearsals are over. I'm ready for my debut!"

By four months, your little one is well on his way to mastering one of the most important of all human skills, the ability to take turns in communicating with others. It all starts with the silly little game of back-and-forth cooing and smiling you do together, called *proto-conversation*, or the first conversation.

And, your infant isn't the only one who's ready for this next chapter of life. I'm sure you're also ready for a little more play . . . and rest. For the past three months, you've unselfishly endured pain, fatigue, and anxiety and you've learned enough to earn a Ph.D. in *Babyology*. So congratulations! All your love and hard work have culminated in this glorious moment. Today, you're one of the most experienced parents on your block . . . and the real fun is just beginning!

~~~~~~~~

Red Flags and Red Alerts: When Should You Call the Doctor?

Fortunately, most colicky babies aren't really ill; they're just "homesick"—struggling to cope with life outside Mama's womb. That's why the 5 S's can be so helpful. But what do you do if the fussing continues despite the 5 S's?

First, check that you're doing the S's correctly. Ask a *Happiest Baby* educator, or review *The Happiest Baby* DVD. If you are doing everything right, call your doctor to have your child examined to make sure he doesn't have a medical problem.

Here's a primer of the ten signs that doctors look for to try to figure out if a child's cries are a sign of frustration or illness. Here, too, are the top ten red-alert conditions your doctor may consider as medical conditions that can cause crying.

TEN RED FLAGS: SIGNS OF A PROBLEM

When you bring your fussy child to the doctor, she will likely ask three questions to help determine if your baby has colic, or something more serious:

1. Is your baby growing well?
2. Is your child normal in all other ways?
3. Does your baby act happy when she's not crying?

If you answered "No" to any of these questions, your doctor will start looking for these red flags and symptoms that indicate a medical problem:

1. Persistent moaning (frequent groans and weak cries)
2. Shrill cry (high-pitched and sharp, unlike your baby's usual cry)
3. Vomiting (more than one ounce per episode; more than five episodes a day; *or any green or yellow vomit*)
4. Change in stool (constipation or diarrhea, especially with blood)
5. Fussing during eating (twisting, arching, crying that begins during or shortly after a feeding)
6. Abnormal temperature (a rectal temperature under 97.5°F or over 100.4°F; under 36.4°C or over 38°C)
7. Irritability (persistent crying with almost no calm periods)
8. Lethargy (a baby sleeping twice as long as usual, acting "out of it," or not sucking well over a twelve-hour period)
9. Bulging soft spot on the head (even when your baby is sitting)
10. Poor weight gain (less than a half ounce a day)

TEN MEDICAL RED ALERTS: ILLNESSES YOUR DOCTOR MAY MENTION

When a doctor examines a fussy baby the first job is to figure out if the crying indicates a serious problem. Food sensitivity or allergy is the only common medical cause of colic. All other problems below occur in less than 1 percent of fussy babies. Below is a list of the top concerns:

1. *Infection: From Ear Infections to Appendicitis*

   You might think the best way to tell if your baby has an infection is to take her temperature, but many sick newborns don't get a fever (some even have low rectal temperatures, below 97.5°F, 36.4°C). If your baby acts lethargic or irritable, call your doctor immediately. She will want to check for:

   EAR INFECTION. Fussy and upset, but rarely swiping at the ears.

   URINE INFECTION. May have smelly urine, but usually don't.

   BRAIN INFECTION (MENINGITIS). Lethargic and/or irritable, vomiting, and a bulging soft spot . . . worsening over 24 hours.

   APPENDICITIS. A hard stomach, poor appetite, and irritability (quite rare in infants).

   INTESTINAL INFECTION. "Stomach flu" that causes vomiting and diarrhea; and the baby may have been in contact with a sick relative or friend.

2. *Intestinal Pain: From Intestinal Blockages to Acid Reflux*

   These problems are the most common medical causes of colic (listed in descending order of frequency):

   FOOD SENSITIVITY/ALLERGY. Five to ten percent of fussy babies have a food problem and improve with a change in

formula or in their mother's diet (if they are breast-fed).
Besides crying, allergies may cause vomiting, diarrhea,
rash, or blood-streaked mucus in the stools. (For more
about food sensitivity/allergies, see chapter 4.)

ACID REFLUX. This burning pain during or after eating causes
less than 1 percent of colic. (For more on acid reflux see
chapter 4.)

INTESTINAL BLOCKAGE. An extremely rare medical emergency.
Babies experience waves of painful spasms plus vomiting, and/or they may stop pooping. With intestinal blockages, the vomit often has a distinct yellow or green tint.

Note: During the first days of life, a breast-fed baby's
spitup may also have a yellow tint (that is the color of colos-
trum). But if your baby's vomit has a yellowish color it's best
to be cautious and immediately call your doctor to make sure
it isn't a sign of something more serious.

3. *Breathing Trouble: From Blocked Nostrils to Oversize*
   Tongues

Blocked nostrils is a common cause of breathing trouble.
Babies are nose breathers except when they're crying. That's
why babies with stuffy noses from allergies or colds get so
frantic.

It's easy to check your baby for a nasal blockage. Place the
tip of your little finger snugly over one of your baby's nostrils,
for a few seconds. She should easily be able to breathe through
the other nostril (you will hear air *wooshing* in and out). Repeat this on the other side.

If your baby gets agitated during the test, the nostril may
be blocked by mucus. Try clearing it with saline or breast
milk drops and a nasal aspirator. And do your best to rid your
home of dust, mold, sprays, perfumes, smoke—including

cigarettes, wood fires, candles, and incense—and anything else that might make her nose congested. However, if the problem continues, call your doctor.

Very rarely, an infant may have trouble breathing because her tongue is too big for her mouth. It literally falls back in the throat and chokes her when she lies on the back. This problem is usually obvious shortly after birth because the tongue is so big it sticks out of the mouth. Fortunately, this issue can usually be improved with a minor surgical procedure.

4. *Increased Brain Pressure*

Too much pressure inside a baby's head, can cause:
- Irritability and crying from a headache
- Vomiting
- An unusual high-pitched cry
- A bulging fontanel (soft spot) even when the baby is seated
- Swollen veins on the forehead
- A head that grows too rapidly (your doctor should measure your baby's head size at every well-baby checkup)
- *Sunset* sign, a big-eyed stare with a crescent of the white of the eye displayed over the colored iris (making the eye look like a setting sun)

If your baby has any of these symptoms, call your doctor immediately.

5. *Skin Pain: A Thread or Hair Twisted Around a Finger, Toe, or Penis*

In years past, sudden sharp screaming in an otherwise calm baby made parents search for an open safety pin inside the diaper. Today, however, parents who hear abrupt, shrill cries should look for a fine hair or thread wrapped tightly around the baby's finger, toe, or penis. This requires immediate medical attention. (Your doctor may treat it by applying a dab of depilatory cream to dissolve the hair.)

6. *Mouth Pain: From Thrush to Teething*

Thrush, a yeast infection in the mouth, is easy to recognize because it causes a milky white residue—that cannot be wiped away—inside the lips and mouth. Sometimes thrush causes a sore mouth, which can make a baby extra fussy. Thrush may also cause a bumpy, red diaper rash, or itchy, red nipples in a breast-feeding mom.

Fortunately it is easy to treat, and recovery is rapid.

You might wonder if teething might cause crying. Teeth are extremely unlikely during the fourth trimester.

7. *Kidney Pain: Blockage of the Urinary System*

A kidney blockage is a very rare cause of crying. Unlike classic colic, which worsens in the evening, kidney pain afflicts children both day and night. And unlike colic, which improves after two or three months, kidney pain usually gets worse over time.

8. *Eye Pain: From Glaucoma to Corneal Abrasion*

Eye pain, also very rare, may come from glaucoma (high pressure inside the eyeball), an accidental scratch of the cornea, or from a tiny, irritating object—such as a cinder or eyelash—stuck under an eyelid. Consider these if your baby has a red, tearing eye.

9. *Overdose: From Excessive Sodium to Vitamin A*

Persistent moaning/crying can result from giving babies excessive sodium (salt). This may occur when a parent mixes formula with too little water. It rarely also occurs during the first few weeks of life if a breast-feeding mom is making very little milk. (Low production can raise the salt level in the milk.) These problems are easy to figure out because the babies are losing weight, not drinking other liquids, and are both irritable and lethargic all day long.

Excess Vitamin A is extremely rare and causes crying only in babies given high doses of supplemental vitamins or fish oil.

Diet supplements, caffeine, chocolate and stimulant Chinese herbs may also pass into the breast milk and cause irritability and crying.

10. Others: From Migraines to Heart Failure

Migraine headaches have been reported to occur more often in children who had colic during infancy. But it is hard to believe that colicky crying is a sign of headache. If that were the cause, why would the crying get better with car rides or vacuum cleaner sounds? (Migraine headaches usually worsen with loud noises.) And why would it peak at six weeks and magically disappear after three or four months?

Other rare conditions causing unstoppable crying include bone fractures, fructose intolerance in babies fed fruit or fruit juice, overactive thyroid, and heart failure. Most of these babies act poorly all day long.

The New Parent's Survival Guide— Ten Key Tips

Behold we count them happy which endure.

James 5:11

Now that we've covered your baby's struggles, let's talk about yours.

Caring for your baby may be the most rewarding work you've ever done, but it may also be the hardest as you cope with hormones, stress, swollen breasts, and fatigue.

As a new parent, you've already noticed that asking five people for advice will get you ten different opinions. (Not that most people even wait for you to ask!) It can be confusing especially if you don't have much "baby experience."

But millions of parents have done this before you; have no doubt that you can be great at it, too!

Here are ten survival tips to help you pass through the challenges of the first few months with a bit more confidence . . . and sanity.

1. *Trust Yourself*

Trust yourself. You know more than you think you do.

Dr. Benjamin Spock

Emily was still in her hospital bed with four-day-old Charlotte. Things were going pretty well, but her confidence as a first-time mom was shaky. "I'm usually such an optimist, yet I've had weird dreams of dropping her and leaving her places. My husband, Roy, joked that he was worried some clueless parent alarm would go off when we tried to take Charlotte home from the hospital!"

Many moms flip back and forth between feeling like a *pro* and like a rookie! Confusing advice given by baby experts (carry more . . . carry less; feed more . . . feed less) can even deepen the angst.

But before you lose confidence remember this: You are part of a continuous chain of successful parents stretching back to the beginning of time! You and your baby have survived because you're descended from the best moms, most protective dads, and strongest children the world has ever seen. You may not know everything, but that's okay . . . billions of parents have done it before you, and they weren't all rocket scientists.

Relax and remember that what your baby needs most is milk and your nourishing love. And what you need is patience, support . . . and maybe a massage every once in a while.

2. *Lower Your Expectations About Knowing What You're Doing*

You'll see. Having a baby is like going to sleep in your own bed and waking up in Zimbabwe!

Sonya to her daughter Denise, a month before
she gave birth to Aidan

One of the biggest surprises after birth is that you don't automatically know how to care for your baby. Beth, a mom of three, quipped, "At the end of my first pregnancy about the only thing I was qualified to do was fill out forms and buy maternity dresses!"

Parenting is easier if you have some experience, but many pregnant couples have never even touched a newborn . . . in their entire lives! (News flash: This has never happened before in human history.)

If people teased you during pregnancy, "Your life will never be the same!" you probably just shrugged it off. Few of us believe *our* baby will be tough. In fact, during pregnancy, your everyday life is so close to normal that it's easy to get lulled into a false sense of security.

Before birth, many women believe that caring for their baby will be just as automatic as pregnancy . . . but as you now know, that couldn't be further from the truth. Before the baby, you can

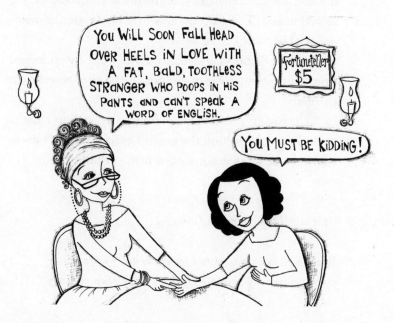

linger in a relaxing tub and think, "I'm ready. I'm on top of this." But after the birth, that long, hot bath you took the month before suddenly starts looking like a far-off Caribbean vacation.

Another shock may be that loving your baby is not as immediate as you expected. Some parents are filled with love the instant they behold their newborn, but not everyone reports feeling smitten right away. And that makes sense; after all, few of us experience love at first sight. But don't worry, just give it a little time to grow. Like the song says, "You can't hurry love."

And one last surprise: After delivery, your brain may change. Memory loss is just one more reminder that your life is temporarily out of your control. One new mom joked, "My best guess is that during the delivery a piece of my brain came out with the placenta."

Many women say that giving birth turned them into complete "boobs"—and in a way they're right. Lactation makes your body awash with prolactin, which, along with the other massive hormonal changes going on inside you, creates a new forgetfulness. (This forgetfulness may help erase the memory of labor pains.)

And this ditziness is made ten times worse by prolonged sleep deprivation. (Read more about *drunk-tired parenting* in chapter 15.)

So be patient and kind to yourself. In a few short months you'll have your feet on the ground again and you'll know your baby better than anyone else in the world!

3. *Accept All the Help You Can Get*

When I moved away from Florida to get my first job, I really enjoyed my new independence. But when my baby was born, I missed my family in a way I had never felt before. Suddenly, I achingly wanted and needed them to be near.

Kathleen, mother of two-month-old Ella Rose

Never in history were parents expected to care for their baby all by themselves. The idea of a nuclear family—one mom and one dad doing it all—may seem normal, but this idea only became routine in the last century. In fact, the nuclear family is one of the craziest—and riskiest—experiments in human history!

For thousands of years, new parents have had bunches of friends and family helping them with housework and baby care . . . and later the couple would return the favor.

Sharon was a work-at-home mom living a thousand miles away from her family with no babysitters or nanny. Sharon was exhausted, but she swore that she would do everything possible to make her kids, Noah and Ariel, happy and healthy. "I feel like an old tomato plant, where the fruit looks plump and delicious even though the plant nourishing it looks scraggly and anemic."

You may think it is totally *cush* to have a nanny, but honestly you're supposed to have five nannies! So, please, don't feel guilty about asking—or paying—for help. Enlist your support team to bring over a frozen casserole, do some cleaning, or watch your baby while you nap. It's okay to lean on them a little—you can pay it back later. The extra help of a niece, nanny, neighbor, or neighbor's older daughter is neither an extravagance nor a sign of failure. *It's the bare minimum help that new parents received since time began.*

4. *Get Your Priorities Straight*

*On the few occasions that my crying baby fell asleep be-
fore I did, I used the time for me! I soaked in a bubble
bath, relaxed with a drink, read a book, and prayed that
she would sleep a little longer.*

Frances Wells Burck, Babysense

I encourage you to get some help, but if you don't have
access to help, don't worry: You'll do fine—as long as you
manage your priorities.

Dedicate this time to caring for the baby, and put off as
many other activities as possible. For example, the week
after having your baby is not the best time to host Aunt
Carol from out of town. As my mother used to say, "Don't
be stupid polite!" A few well-wishers are fine, but only if
they're healthy and helpful. Visitors who can't cook or clean
take up your precious time and, what's worse, they carry
germs into your home. People may call you paranoid but, in
truth, having a new baby is the best reason for being over-
protective.

To show your appreciation to everyone who calls, leave a
sweet announcement on your phone, telling everyone the
baby's key statistics and announcing that you won't be returning calls for a few weeks. Of course, you can call back
sooner, but this gives you some breathing room, in case you'd
rather focus on higher priorities—such as soaking in a hot
tub.

Rest: The Essential Vitamin for New Parents

Sometimes the most urgent and vital thing you can do . . . is take a nap.

Ashleigh Brilliant

As teenagers, we were "dying" to stay up all night. Now, we're "dying" if we have to stay up all night! The extreme fatigue that goes along with being a new parent can distort our view of the world like a fun-house mirror, leaving us feeling anxious, depressed, irritable, and inept. (Some countries actually torture people by waking them up every time they fall asleep!)

So, nap when your baby does, sleep when your mom comes, and—*however you do it*—get some rest!

5. *Be Flexible*

You just have to accept that some days you're the pigeon and some days you're the statue.

Roger Anderson

There are times in life when an unwillingness to compromise is admirable—but after becoming a new parent isn't one of them. I think the official bumper sticker for all new parents should read, *Be flexible—or die!*

Part of the privilege of parenting is choosing how you want to raise your child. But it's also important for you to be able to throw your expectations out the window and start all over again when things are going haywire.

If you enjoyed being organized, on time, and having a spotless house, this new flexibility may require practice—

and deep breathing. Now is the time to chuck your to-do list for a few months; accept that your clock has been temporarily transformed from a tool to a wall decoration; and know that, for a while, day and night will cease to have any true relevance.

You've "bought your ticket" for this roller coaster so let go and open yourself to the marvel, awe, and exhilaration of one of the greatest adventures of life!

6. *Know Thyself: How Do Your Baby's Cries Make You Feel?*

When your baby screams, can you calmly think, "He must be having a bad day"? Or does your anxiety and frustration bubble up: "I must be doing something wrong!" or, "I don't deserve to be a mother!" Or even, "Who the hell does she think she is?"

A baby's screams can have a powerful effect on the mind, triggering a flood of upsetting feelings from the past. You may suddenly remember voices of criticism, and ridicule directed at you long ago. And you may find yourself getting angry or defensive. Of course, all this isn't rational. Your baby is much too young to criticize you. But fatigue and stress can fool your mind and make these innocent cries feel like stinging attacks.

Please don't judge yourself. This is all a normal part of being a new parent. When emotions well up inside, take the opportunity to be brave and share your feelings with your spouse or someone else who truly cares about you. The more you discuss past pains and current fears, the better you'll be able to uncouple your baby's cries from old stresses and traumas.

7. *Don't Rock the Cradle Too Hard: Frustration, and Child Abuse*

David felt a wave of anger blowing across him like a hot wind. After weeks of colicky screaming by both of his twins,

Sam and Ben, he snapped and punched his hand through a door. "I was so frustrated and exhausted I couldn't control myself. I would never hurt my boys, but for the first time in my life I understood how even a good parent could be driven to such desperation."

Few things make us feel better than being able to quickly soothe our baby's screams. And when everything we do fails, few things make us feel worse.

Remember, your baby can scream louder than a vacuum cleaner. No wonder it's so painful when she's cuddled on your shoulder, blasting right next to your ear. The sound of your baby's cry sets off a "red alert" inside your own nervous system, making your heart race, your skin cringe, and creating an urgent desire to stop it. Crying can be especially difficult when coupled with fatigue, depression, financial stress, pain, hormonal chaos, family conflict, and a history of being abused.

These combined forces can push even a loving parent over the edge into the dark abyss of abuse. A mild-mannered father told me his daughter's cries started to "get to him" in the middle of the night and he found himself rocking her cradle *a little too hard*. "I felt so incompetent, like such a terrible parent. My little Marlo was so unhappy, yet nothing I did seemed to help."

No matter how desperate you feel, remember that there's a *huge* difference between feelings and actions. It's totally fine to make silly jokes about leaving your baby on someone's doorstep if you're feeling overwhelmed . . . just don't do it.

And if you're getting close to the breaking point:

• Lighten your workload and get some assistance cleaning the house and watching the baby.
• Do something physical to vent your energy: Dig a hole, hammer nails, beat the sofa, scream into a pillow, take a run.

- Talk to someone: a friend, a relative, or the National Child Abuse Hotline at 1-800-4-A-CHILD (1-800-422-4453). It has counselors available every day, all day.

8. *Keep Your Sense of Humor Handy*

He who laughs . . . lasts!

Mary Pettibone Poole

There are times when parenthood seems like nothing but feeding the mouth that bites you.

Peter De Vries

The only normal families are the ones you don't know very well.

Joe Ancis

Babies are always more trouble than you thought . . . and more wonderful.

Charles Osgood

It's not easy for me to take my problems one at a time when they refuse to get in line.

Ashleigh Brilliant

Raising a child is a constant series of tasks and challenges. You don't want to make mistakes, but you will. Remember, perfection is only found in the dictionary. So, let go of dignity, forget organization, be gentle with yourself . . . and laugh!

Laughter is exactly what this doctor orders. Rent some funny movies or watch reruns of *Friends*. Try imagining Kim Kardashian burping her baby and getting a giant spitup down her back. Laugh at your hair, laugh at your baby, laugh at your messy house. Laugh when your little darling's diaper leaks on your sofa. And laugh at the fact that you're now one of those women—heatedly discussing burping and the color of her baby's poop—who you used to avoid at parties.

9. *Take Care of Your Spouse (S/he Just Might Come in Handy)*

When Cheryl and Jeff's second child Curtis was four weeks old, Jeff said, "We haven't even had sex once yet." Cheryl shot back, "What do you expect? Every sexual part of my body is either oozing, throbbing, or bruised!"

Taking care of a new baby is so demanding and time-consuming that it's easy to feel like you're slaving away at 110 percent effort (usually true) and your partner is only chipping in 70 percent (usually false).

The truth is, being new parents is totally a joint effort. There is so much to do that the only way to get it all done— and still be friends—is to work as a team.

Think about it from your baby's perspective. Her world balances on the two of you. She would never want to hear you say "Baby, I gave up everything for you. I even put you ahead of your father/mother." In fact, if your infant could, she'd sit you down and say, "Don't worry about me. I'm fine, but I'm really gonna need you two later on. So, go have some fun, see a movie, but please take care of yourselves!"

Caring for your baby is a big job; but you still have to make time to give each other a little TLC. Support and adore, nurture and caress each other. Take walks, give each other massages, back scratches, and gentle intimacy. Don't take your partner for granted and never go to bed angry. Cut each other some extra slack and avoid judgments and harsh criti-cisms.

These first months are the hardest part of the first year, but the great news is, if you work as a team, your relationship will emerge stronger than ever.

To Dads: Appreciate Your Wife, the Great Goddess of Creation

Mothers are great heroes! When it comes to making babies, we men chip in a few sperm while our wives essentially pull a wagon from Alaska to the Gulf of Mexico. In fact, except for your twenty-three chromosomes, every single molecule of your baby was individually carried through your wife's body. It's almost as if each cell should carry a little tag that reads, *Inspected by Mom*.

While you spent the past nine months going about your life in a fairly normal way, your partner has been stretched in a surreal kind

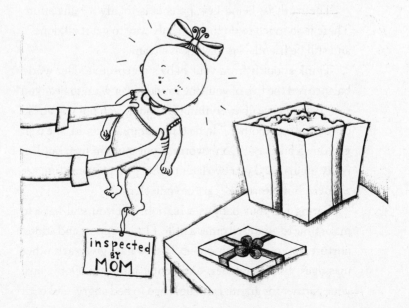

of mind-body taffy pull. Let's face it, any guy who has watched his wife give birth knows the real truth about who is the weaker sex.

And, after your child is born, your wife has another awesome responsibility. While you get to go to work, she's at home dealing with leaking breasts, sore nipples, losing that extra thirty pounds, and a frantic, red-faced person yelling at her for no good reason . . . and all this with little or no training.

And then there's sex (or no sex)! When the milk comes, your wife may look like she just had a boob job. And you may crave intimacy after abstaining for the last weeks/months. But new moms often have "pelvic exhaustion" and may not be feeling very erotic. (Remember, those boobies have to be shared with the baby.)

Your wife needs your attention, support, and tenderness more than ever. Bring home flowers, change some diapers, and give her a break to go out with friends. That's the type of "child support" she really needs!

Note: It's no accident that one of the best predictors of breast-feeding success and avoiding depression is a spouse's support.

To Moms: Appreciate Your Husband, the Man Who Put the *Us* in *Uterus*

Okay, Mom, it's true: You've had to do all the "heavy lifting" so far, and you barely have the time to pee—but it's not easy being a new dad, either. Remember, your husband has big expectations of himself, too. Most guys feel a huge pressure to go into the world and compete to provide for their families.

Even if your partner is quiet, don't think he doesn't feel things as deeply as you do. Many new dads feel as nervous handling their infants as they did asking a girl to the prom. Men shown crying babies have the same sharp increase in sweating, heart rate, and blood pressure.

So be patient with your sweetie. Be available if he needs you, but don't rescue him right away when he's fumbling around trying to get the hang of swaddling or calming your baby with the 5 S's. He'll sense your confidence in him and feel great when he can do it on his own.

10. *Don't Ignore Depression: The Uninvited Guest*

As shocking as it sounds, 10 to 40 percent of new moms experience unhappy feelings intruding upon their joy in the weeks after giving birth. They notice themselves becoming more anxious, tearful, worried, or exhausted—yet unable to sleep—all of these may be early signs of postpartum depression (PPD).

Women can experience three different levels of depression:

BABY BLUES: Mild weepiness, anxiety, and insomnia.

TRUE POSTPARTUM DEPRESSION: A bruising, more debilitating type of grief.

POSTPARTUM PSYCHOSIS: A severe and rare condition that includes hallucinations, incoherent statements, and bizarre behavior.

Note: Experts have long speculated that the huge hormone shifts that occur during childbirth trigger PPD. But I have my doubts about this theory because it fails to explain why PPD can: a) start months after delivery; b) occur in moms who adopt babies; c) affect many new dads.

The Baby Blues

The baby blues usually start during the few weeks after the baby is born and last from days to weeks. No one knows exactly why it occurs, but the sadness can be made worse by other stresses—such as sleep deprivation and infant fussing.

The blues are so common that many doctors consider them a normal part of parenting. Nonetheless, the unanticipated angst, fear, and sorrow can be very distressing.

Feeling dejected and rejected, Sarah called me one evening. She had it with her four-week-old. Sarah said, "Julie's fussy and demanding all the time; I feel robbed of my joy. I dread her crying because I never know if it will last two minutes or two hours! And on top of that, I'm a light sleeper and so attuned to her cry that I rarely sleep more than a catnap.

"I'm anxious, exhausted . . . falling apart. My babysitter acts so calmly around Julie and I couldn't help but feel that I was making my baby worse with my awkward attempts at calming her."

I asked Sarah and Tom to come in so I could teach them the 5 S's. I thought much of Sarah's problem might stem from exhaustion, but I was also concerned about early signs of depression. At the end of our meeting, I encouraged Sarah to make an appointment with a psychiatrist, just in case the techniques didn't help. Fortunately, Sarah quickly mastered the skills and saw a dramatic improvement in Julie's calming and sleep. As Julie slept more, Sarah did, too . . . and she began to feel like a better mom. "Within a week," she said, "I felt the darkness lift and my life turn around. Yesterday, I calmed my little baby in less than two minutes. I was so proud!"

Note: Although we use the term *depression,* many women suffer much more from panic and fear than sadness.

True Postpartum Depression

> *My whole world suddenly turned black. My emotions jumped from guilt to despair to such utter anxiety that I thought I would either jump out of my skin or lose my*

> *mind. I imagined injuring myself so I could be taken to*
> *the hospital and rescued from this overwhelming burden.*
> *I felt like I was being punished for thinking I could be a*
> *good mother. I felt like I didn't deserve to have a*
> *child . . . and I cried for hours.*
>
> Louisa, mother of three-week-old Georgia

If mild sadness after birth is called the *baby blues,* more severe depression should be called the *baby black and blues,* because it is a bruising assault on a woman's psychological health. During the first weeks of what should be the greatest bliss of their lives, about 10 percent of moms experience strong feelings of anxiety and sorrow.

These symptoms can occur at any time after delivery and last from weeks to many months . . . or longer. They are made worse by other stresses, including infant crying, exhaustion, pain, lack of support, financial pressures, family problems, and so forth. PPD can strike up to 50 percent of new moms in high risk situations.

Exhaustion mixed with a baby's screams may trigger a flood of painful memories, such as being yelled at in anger or ridicule. Crashing waves of emotion can make moms feel like they're drowning in sadness, shame, fear, and hopelessness. No matter what words of support her loved ones offer, she may think it's impossible for them to really understand how she feels. And, as Louisa experienced, depression can cause victims to fantasize about hurting themselves or their babies.

This black hole sucks away a woman's optimism and confidence. Yet the accompanying shame and isolation leads most women to keep their suffering a secret from their family, friends, and doctors.

If you are feeling like this, please know that you're not alone . . . or at fault! *Depression is a medical illness!* And, you are no more responsible—or deserving of guilt—than people who suffer from allergies.

Please reach out for help!

Your doctor may recommend a support group, exercise, more sunlight (or a daylight intensity home lamp), better diet (extra vitamin D and omega-3 fatty acids), antidepressant medicine, hypnosis, or counseling. (Unfortunately, there's no evidence that powdered placenta capsules are any more effective than placebo.) And use the 5 S's (including rumbly sound all night) to boost your baby's sleep . . . and yours. Often just a few nights of better rest can make a big difference in your outlook.

Note: Severe depression may also be caused by a sudden drop in your thyroid level. Make sure your doctor checks you for this very treatable condition.

For help with any level of postpartum depression, contact:

Postpartum Support International:

800-944-4PPD or www.postpartum.net

Depression After Delivery:

www.depressionafterdelivery.com

Postpartum Psychosis

This terrible reaction occurs in about one in one thousand women, usually within two weeks of delivery. Typically, these distraught new mothers hear voices calling them names or telling them to do horrible things. They also become obsessive and preoccupied with bizarre, repetitive acts; refuse to eat; and become frantically active and extremely confused.

If you think you—or someone you know—may be suffering from this serious condition, seek medical help immediately.

Postpartum psychosis is treatable, but it's an absolute medical emergency!

BIBLIOGRAPHY

Below is a listing of sources for many of the key research findings noted in the book.

Introduction. Ancient Secrets About Crying Babies

Parmelee AH. Remarks on receiving the C. Anderson Aldrich Award. *Pediatrics.* 1977; 59: 389–95.

Konner M. Hunter-gatherer infancy: The !Kung and others. In: Hewlett BS and Lamb ME, eds. *Hunter-Gatherer Childhoods: Evolutionary, Developmental and Cultural Perspectives.* New Brunswick, NJ: Aldine Transaction; 2005:19–64.

Barr RG, Konner M, et al. Crying in !Kung San infants: A test of the cultural specificity hypothesis. *Dev Med Child Neurol.* 1991; 33: 601–10.

Liedloff J. *The Continuum Concept: In Search of Happiness Lost.* New York, NY: Da Capo Press; 1986.

Chapter 1. Babies: A New Insight

Brazelton TB. Crying in infancy. *Pediatrics.* 1962; 4: 579–88.

Barr RG, et al. Effectiveness of educational materials designed to change knowledge and behaviors regarding crying and shaken-baby syndrome in mothers of newborns: A randomized, controlled trial. *Pediatrics.* 2009; 123: 972–80.

Mayer J. The experiment. *New Yorker.* July 11, 2005. http://www.newyorker.com/magazine/2005/07/11/the-experiment-3.

St. James-Roberts I, Halil T. Infant crying patterns in the first year: Normal community and clinical findings. *J Child Psychol Psychiatry.* 1991; 32: 951–68.

Konner, M. Hunter-gatherer infancy: The !Kung and others. In: Hewlett BS and Lamb ME, eds. *Hunter-Gatherer Childhoods: Evolutionary, Developmental and Cultural Perspectives.* New Brunswick, NJ: Aldine Transaction; 2005:19–64.

Chapter 2. Crying: Our Infants' Ancient Survival Tool

Anisfeld E, et al. Does infant carrying promote attachment? An experimental study of the effects of increased physical contact on the development of attachment. *Child Dev.* 1990; 61: 1617–27.

Lorenz K. *Studies in Animal and Human Behavior.* Cambridge, MA: Harvard University Press; 1971.

Frodi AM, et al. Fathers' and mothers' responses to infant smiles and cries. *Infant Behav Dev.* 1978; 1: 187–98.

Levitzky S, Cooper R. Infant colic syndrome: maternal fantasies of aggression and infanticide. *Clin Pediatr (Phila).* 2000; 39: 395–400.

Papousek M, von Hofacker N. Persistent crying in early infancy: a nontrivial condition of risk for the developing mother-infant relationship. *Child Care Health Dev.* 1998; 24: 395–424.

Ross LE, McLean LM. Anxiety disorders during pregnancy and

the postpartum period: A systematic review. *J Clin Psychiatry.* 2006; 67: 1285–98.

Maxted AE, et al. Infant colic and maternal depression. *Infant Ment Health J.* 2005; 26: 56–68.

Radesky J, et al. Inconsolable infant crying and maternal postpartum depressive symptoms. *Pediatrics.* 2013; 131: 1–8.

Acebo C, Thoman EB. Crying as social behavior. *Infant Ment Health J.* 1992; 13: 67–82.

Gustafson GE, Harris, KL. Women's responses to young infants' cries. *Dev Psychol.* 1990; 26: 144–52.

Wasz-Hockert O, et al. The identification of some specific meanings in infant vocalization. *Experientia.* 1964; 20: 154–56.

Wasz-Hockert O, et al. *The Infant Cry: A Spectrographic and Auditory Analysis.* Clinics in Developmental Medicine (Rep. No. 29). London: Spastics International Medical Publications; 1968.

Dunston Baby Language website. http://www.dunstanbaby.com.

Lester B, Barr R, eds. Colic and Excessive Crying. Report of the 105th Ross Conference on Pediatric Research; 1997.

Barr R, St. James-Roberts I, Keefe M, eds. New Evidence on Unexplained Early Infant Crying: Its Origins, Nature, and Management. Johnson and Johnson Pediatric Institute, Pediatric Round Table; 2001.

Chapter 3. The Dreaded Colic: A "CRYsis" for the Whole Family

Brazelton TB. Crying in infancy. *Pediatrics.* 1962; 4: 579–88.

St. James-Roberts I, Halil T: Infant crying patterns in the first year: Normal community and clinical findings. *J Child Psychol Psychiatry.* 1991; 32: 951–68.

Barr RG, et al. Effectiveness of educational materials designed to change knowledge and behaviors regarding crying and shaken-baby syndrome in mothers of newborns: a randomized, controlled trial. *Pediatrics.* 2009; 123: 972–80.

Wessel MA, et al. Paroxysmal fussing in infancy, sometimes called "colic." *Pediatrics.* 1954; 14: 421–34.

Barr R, St. James-Roberts I, Keefe M, eds. New Evidence on Unexplained Early Infant Crying: Its Origins, Nature, and Management. Johnson and Johnson Pediatric Institute, Pediatric Round Table; 2001.

National Center on Shaken Baby Syndrome website. http:// dontshake.org.

Clifford TJ, et al. Infant colic: Empirical evidence of the absence of an association with source of early infant nutrition. *Arch Pediatr Adolesc Med.* 2002; 156: 1123–28.

Barr RG, et al. Crying patterns in preterm infants. *Dev Med Child Neurol.* 1996; 38: 345–55.

Pierce PP. Delayed onset of "three months" colic in premature infants. *Arch Pediatr Adolesc Med.* 1948; 75: 190.

Paradise JL: Maternal and other factors in the etiology of infantile colic. *JAMA.* 1966; 197: 123–31.

Hubbard FOA, van IJzendoorn MH. Maternal unresponsiveness and infant crying across the first 9 months: A longitudinal study. *Infant Behav Dev.* 1991; 14: 299–312.

Chapter 4. The Top Five Colic Theories, and Why They're (Mostly) Wrong

Illingsworth R. The 3-months colic. *Arch Dis Child.* 1954; 29: 165–74.

Danielsson B, Hwang CP. Treatment of infantile colic with surface active substance (simethicone). *Acta Paediatr Scand.* 1985; 74: 446–50.

Metcalf T, et al. Simethicone in the treatment of infantile colic. *Pediatrics.* 1994; 94: 29–34.

Mennella JA, et al. Prenatal and postnatal flavor learning by human infants. *Pediatrics.* 2001; 107: E88.

Jakobsson I, Lindberg T. Cow's milk proteins cause colic in

breast-fed infants: A double-blind crossover study. *Pediatrics.* 1983; 71: 268–71.

Lucassen P, et al. Effectiveness of treatments for infantile colic: Systematic review. *BMJ.* 1998; 16: 1563–69.

Forsythe BW. Colic and the effect of changing formulas. *J Pediatr.* 1989; 115: 521–26.

Santos IS, et al. Maternal caffeine consumption and infant nighttime waking: Prospective cohort study. *Pediatrics.* 2012; 129: 860–68.

Liebman WM. Infantile colic association with lactose and milk intolerance. *JAMA.* 1981; 245: 732–33.

Barr RG, et al. Carbohydrate change has no effect on infant crying behavior: A randomized controlled study. *Am J Dis Child.* 1987; 141: 391.

Sanz Y. Gut microbiota and probiotics in maternal and infant health. *Am J Clin Nutr.* 2011; 94: Suppl. 6.

Embleton N, Berrington JE. Probiotics reduce the risk of necrotising enterocolitis (NEC) in preterm infants. *Am J Clin Nutri.* 2013; 18: 219–20.

Savino F et al. Lactobacillus reuteri DSM 17938 in infantile colic: A randomized, double-blind, placebo-controlled trial. *Pediatrics.* 2010; 126: e526.

Kim Chau K, et al. Probiotics for infantile colic: A randomized, double-blind, placebo-controlled trial investigating Lactobacillus reuteri DSM 17938. *J Pediatr.* 2015; 166: 74–78.

Sung V, et al. Probiotics to prevent or treat excessive infant crying: Systematic review and meta-analysis. *JAMA Pediatr.* 2013; 167: 1150–57.

Sung V, et al. Treating infant colic with the probiotic Lactobacillus reuteri: Double blind, placebo controlled randomised trial. *BMJ.* 2014; 348: g2107.

Rhoads JM et al. Altered fecal microflora and increased fecal calprotectin in infants with colic. *J Pediatr.* 2009; 155: 823–28.

Heine R, et al. Role of gastro-oesophageal reflux in infant irritability. *Arch Dis Child.* 1995; 73: 121–25.

de Boissieu D, et al. Distinct features of upper gastrointestinal endoscopy in the newborn. *J Pediatr Gastroenterol Nutr.* 1994; 18: 334–38.

Orenstein SR, et al. Multicenter, double-blind, randomized, placebo-controlled trial assessing the efficacy and safety of proton pump inhibitor Lansoprazole in infants with symptoms of gastroesophageal reflux disease. *J Pediatr.* 2009; 154: 514–20.

Menchise AN, Cohen MB. Acid-reducing agents in infants and children: Friend or foe? *JAMA Pediatr.* 2014; 168: 888–90.

Hassall, E. Over-prescription of acid-suppressing medications in infants: how it came about, why it's wrong, and what to do about it. *J Pediatr.* 2012; 160: 193–98.

Vandenplas Y, et al: Continuous 24-hour esophageal pH monitoring in 285 asymptomatic infants 0–15 months old. *J Pediatr Gastroenterol Nutr.* 1987; 6: 220–24.

Eom, Chun-Sick, et al. Use of acid-suppressive drugs and risk of pneumonia: a systematic review and meta-analysis. *CMAJ.* 2011; 183: 310–19.

Rosen R, et al. Changes in gastric and lung microflora with acid suppression: Acid suppression and bacterial growth. *JAMA Pediatr.* 2014; 168: 932–37.

Giuliano C, et al. Are proton pump inhibitors associated with the development of community-acquired pneumonia? A meta-analysis. *Expert Rev Clin Pharmacol.* 2012; 5: 337–44.

Hennessy, Sean, et al. Cisapride and ventricular arrhythmia. *Br J Clin Pharmacol.* 2008; 66: 375–85.

St. James-Roberts I, et al. Clinical, developmental, and social aspects of infant crying and colic. *Early Dev Parenting.* 1995; 4: 177–89.

Fox, NA, Polak, CP. The possible contribution of temperament to understanding the origins and consequences of persistent and excessive crying. In: Barr R, St. James-Roberts I, Keefe M, eds. New Evidence on Unexplained Early Infant Crying: Its Origins, Nature, and Management. Johnson and Johnson Pediatric Institute, Pediatric Round Table; 2001: 25–42.

Barr RG, et al. Feeding and temperament as determinants of early infant crying/fussing behavior. *Pediatrics.* 1989; 84: 514–21.

Lehtonen L, et al. Temperament and sleeping patterns in colicky infants during the first year of life. *J Dev Behav Pediatr.* 1994; 15: 416–20.

Stifter CA, Braungart J. Infant colic: A transient condition with no apparent effects. *J Appl Dev Psychol.* 1992; 13: 447–62.

Papousek M, et al. Persistent crying and parenting: Search for a butterfly in a dynamic system. *Early Dev Parenting.* 1995; 4: 209–24.

Chapter 5. The True Cause of Colic: The Missing Fourth Trimester

U.S. Department of Labor. *Infant Care.* Washington, DC: US Government Printing Office; 1914. Revised 1929.

Bell SM, Ainsworth MDS. Infant crying and maternal responsiveness. *Child Dev.* 1972; 43: 1171–90.

Wasz-Hockert O, et al. The identification of some specific meanings in infant vocalization. *Experientia.* 1964; 20: 154–56.

Barr RG, Konner M, et al. Crying in !Kung San infants: A test of the cultural specificity hypothesis. *Dev Med Child Neurol.* 1991; 33: 601–10.

Chapter 6. The Fourth Trimester: The Woman Who Mistook Her Baby for a Horse

Parmelee AH. Remarks on receiving the C. Anderson Aldrich Award. *Pediatrics.* 1977; 59: 389–95.

Liu, Dong, et al. Maternal care, hippocampal synaptogenesis and cognitive development in rats. *Nat Neurosci.* 2000; 3: 799–806.

Barr RG, Konner M, et al. Crying in !Kung San infants: A test of

the cultural specificity hypothesis. *Dev Med Child Neurol.* 1991;
33: 601–10.

Chapter 7. The Key to Happy Babies: The Calming Reflex and the *5 S's*

9 Newborn reflexes. *Parenting* website. http://www.parenting
.com/gallery/newborn-reflexes.

Period of PURPLE crying. National Center on Shaken Baby
Syndrome website. http://www.dontshake.org/purpleprogram.

Turgeon-O'Brien, H, et al. Nutritive and nonnutritive sucking
habits: a review. *ASDC J Dent Child.* 1995; 63: 321–27.

Adler M. Promoting Maternal Child Health by Teaching Parents
to Calm Fussy Infants. Presented at the CDC CityMatCH
Urban MCH Leadership Conference. Denver, CO; August 28,
2007.

Pennsylvania Department of Health. Cries to Smiles. Harrisburg,
PA: Pennsylvania Department of Health. Breast-feeding
Awareness and Support Group; 2007.

Data Summary of *Happiest Baby on the Block* Retrospective Post-
Test Surveys. Southeastern Arizona Behavioral Health Services.
Evaluation Research and Development Team (ERAD); 2007–8
and 2008–9.

Chapter 8. 1st *S*: Swaddling—A Feeling of Pure "WRAPture"

Bakwin H. Loneliness in infants. *Am J Dis Child.* 1942; 63: 30–40.

Bakwin H. Emotional deprivation in infants. *J Pediatr.* 1949;
35: 512–21.

Crying baby less than three months old. American Academy of
Pediatrics website. http://www.healthychildren.org/English
/tips-tools/Symptom-Checker/Pages/Crying-Baby-Less
-Than-3-Months-Old.aspx.

Jana LA, Shu J. *Heading Home with Your Newborn.* New York, NY:
American Academy of Pediatrics; 2005.

American Academy of Pediatrics website.
http://www2.aap.org/sections/scan/practicingsafety/toolkit
_resources/module1/swadling.pdf

Task force on sudden infant death syndrome for a safe infant
sleeping environment SIDS and other sleep-related infant
deaths: Expansion of recommendations. *Pediatrics.* 2011;
128: e1341–67.

SIDS and Kids website. http://www.sidsandkids.org. "Safe
Wrapping: Guide for Safe Wrapping of Young Babies."

Swaddling: IHDI position statement. International Hip Dysplasia
Institute website. http://www.hipdysplasia.org/For-Physicians
/Pediatricians/default.aspx.

Thach B. Does swaddling decrease or increase the risk for sudden
infant death syndrome? *J Pediatr.* 2009; 155: 461–62.

Ahluwalia IB, et al. Why do women stop breastfeeding? Findings
from the Pregnancy Risk Assessment and Monitoring System.
Pediatrics. 2005; 116: 1408–12.

Li R, et al. Why mothers stop breastfeeding: Mothers' self-
reported reasons for stopping during the 1st year. *Pediatrics.*
2008; 122: s69–s76.

Catherine N, et al. Should we do more to get the word out? Causes
of, responses to, and consequences of crying and colic in
popular parenting magazines. *J Dev Behav Pediatr.* 2005;
26: 14–23.

Barr RG, et al. Age-related incidence curve of hospitalized Shaken
Baby Syndrome cases: Convergent evidence for crying as a trigger
to shaking. *Child Abuse Negl.* 2006; 30: 7–16.

Talvik I, et al. Shaken baby syndrome and a baby's cry. *Acta
Paediatr.* 2008; 97: 782–85.

Willinger, M. et al. Factors associated with caregivers' choice of
infant sleep position, 1994–98: The national infant sleep position
study. *JAMA.* 2000; 283: 2135–42.

Von Kohorn I, et al. Influence of prior advice and beliefs of mothers

on infant sleep position. *Arch Pediatr Adolesc Med.* 2010;
164: 363–69.

St. James-Roberts I, Halil T: Infant crying patterns in the first year:
Normal community and clinical findings. *J Child Psychol
Psychiatry.* 1991; 32: 951–68.

Sutphen J. Is it colic or is it gastroesophageal reflux? *J Pediatr
Gastroenterol Nutr.* 2001; 33: 110–11.

Gaffney KF, Henry LL. Identifying risk factors for postpartum
tobacco use. *J Nurs Scholarsh.* 2007; 39: 126–32.

Gaffney KF, et al. Mothers' reflections about infant irritability and
postpartum tobacco use. *Birth.* 2008; 35: 66–72.

2004 Sleep in America Poll Final Report. National Sleep Foundation.
March 2004. http://www.sleepfoundation.org/sites
/default/files/2004SleepPollFinalReport.pdf.

Taheri S, et al. Short sleep duration is associated with reduced
leptin, elevated ghrelin, and increased body mass index (BMI).
Sleep. 2004; 27: A146–47.

Ponsonby, A, et al. Factors potentiating the risk of Sudden Infant
Death Syndrome associated with the Prone Position. *N Engl J
Med.* 1993; 329: 377–82.

Blair PS, et al. Hazardous cosleeping environments and risk factors
amenable to change: Case-control study of SIDS in south west
England. *BMJ.* 2009; 339: b3666.

SIDS and Kids website. http://www.sidsandkids.org.

Wilson CA, Taylor BJ, Laing RM, et al. Clothing and bedding and
its relevance to sudden infant death syndrome: further results
from the New Zealand Cot Death Study. *J Paediatr Child
Health.* 1994; 30: 506–12.

McDonnell E, Moon RY. Infant deaths and injuries associated with
wearable blankets, swaddle wraps, and swaddling. *J Pediatr.*
2014; 164: 1152–66.

Rechtman LR, et al. Sofas and infant mortality. *Pediatrics.* 2014;
134: e1293–e1300.

Li DK, et al. Infant sleeping position and the risk of sudden infant death syndrome in California, 1997–2000. *Am J Epidemiol.* 2003; 157: 446–55.

Vennemann MM, et al. Sleep environment risk factors for sudden infant death syndrome: The German sudden infant death syndrome study. *Pediatrics.* 2009; 123: 1162–70.

Oden RP, et al. Swaddling: Will it get babies onto their backs for sleep? *Clin Pediatr.* 2012; 51: 254–59.

Schoendorf KC, Kiely JL. Relationship of sudden infant death syndrome to maternal smoking during and after pregnancy. *Pediatrics.* 1992; 90: 905–8.

Liebrechts-Akkerman G, et al. Postnatal parental smoking: An important risk factor for SIDS. *Eur J Pediatr.* March 2011. doi: 10.1007/s00431-011-1433-6.

Gaffney KF, Henry LL. Identifying risk factors for postpartum tobacco use. *J Nurs Scholarsh.* 2007; 39: 126–32.

Gaffney K, et al. Mothers' Reflections about infant irritability and Postpartum Tobacco Use. *Birth.* 2008; 35: 66–72.

Vennemann, MM, et al. Does Breastfeeding Reduce the Risk of Sudden Infant Death Syndrome? *Pediatrics.* 2009; 123: e406–10.

Hauck FR et al. Breastfeeding and reduced risk of sudden infant death syndrome: A meta-analysis. *Pediatrics.* 2011; 128: 103–10.

Ahluwalia IB, et al. Why do women stop breastfeeding? Findings from the pregnancy risk assessment and monitoring system. *Pediatrics.* 2005; 116: 1408–12.

Dennis CL, McQueen K. The relationship between infant-feeding outcomes and postpartum depression: A qualitative systematic review. *Pediatrics.* 2009; 23: e736–51.

Li R, et al. Why mothers stop breastfeeding: Mothers' self-reported reasons for stopping during the 1st year, *Pediatrics* 2008; 122: s69–s76.

Ueda T, et al. Influence of psychological stress on suckling-induced pulsatile oxytocin release. *Obstet Gynecol.* 1994; 84: 259–62.

Riordan JM, Nichols FH. A descriptive study of lactation mastitis in long-term breastfeeding women. *J Hum Lact.* 1990; 6: 53–58.

Pauli-Pott U, et al. Infants with "colic": Mothers' perspectives on the crying problem. *J Psychosom Res.* 2000; 48: 125–32.

MacDonald MG, Mullett MD, Seshia MMK., eds. *Avery's Neonatology: Pathophysiology and Management of the Newborn.* 6th ed. Philadelphia: Lippincott Williams and Wilkins; 2005.

Pennsylvania Department of Health. *Cries to Smiles.* Harrisburg, PA: Pennsylvania Department of Health, Breastfeeding Awareness and Support Group; 2007.

Mohrbacher N. Rethinking swaddling. *Int J Childbirth Educ.* 2010; 25: 7–10.

Giacoman SL. Hunger and motor restraint on arousal and visual attention in the infant. *Child Dev.* 1971; 42: 605–14.

Gerard CM, Harris KA, Thach BT. Physiologic studies on swaddling: An ancient child care practice, which may promote the supine position for infant sleep. *J Pediatr.* 2002; 141: 398–404.

Lipton E, et al. Swaddling, a child care practice: Historical, cultural and experimental observations. *Pediatrics.* 1965; 35 (Sup): 521–67.

Franco P, et al. Influence of swaddling on sleep and arousal characteristics of healthy infants. *Pediatrics.* 2005; 115: 1307–11.

Richardson HL, et al. Minimizing the risks of sudden infant death syndrome: to swaddle or not to swaddle? *J Pediatr.* 2009; 155: 475–81.

Williams SM, et al. Sudden infant death syndrome: Insulation from bedding and clothing and its effect modifiers. *Int J Epidemiol.* 1996; 25: 366–75.

Ponsonby AL, et al. The Tasmanian SIDS case-control study: Univariable and multivariable risk factor analysis. *Paediatr Perinat Epidemiol.* 1995; 9: 256–72.

Ponsonby AL, et al. Thermal environment and sudden infant death syndrome: case-control study. *BMJ*. 1992; 304: 277–83.

Gestel JPJ van, et al. Risks of ancient practices in modern times. *Pediatrics*. 2002; 110: e78.

Beal S, Porter C. Sudden infant death syndrome related to climate. *Acta Paediatr Scand*. 1991; 80: 278–87.

Cheng TL, Partridge JC. Effect of bundling and high environmental temperature on neonatal body temperature. *Pediatrics*. 1993; 92: 238–40.

Grover G, et al. The effects of bundling on infant temperature. *Pediatrics*. 1994; 94: 669–73.

Tsogt B, et al. Can traditional care influence thermoregulation? A prospective controlled study of the effects of swaddling on infants' thermal balance in a Mongolian winter. 9th SIDS Conference; June 1–4, 2006.

Richardson H, et al. Sleep position alters arousal processes maximally at the high-risk age for sudden infant death syndrome, *J Sleep Res*. 2008; 17: 450–57.

Richardson HL, et al. Minimizing the risks of sudden infant death syndrome: To swaddle or not to swaddle? *J Pediatr*. 2009; 155: 475–81.

Richardson HL, et al. Influence of swaddling experience on spontaneous arousal patterns and autonomic control in sleeping infants. *J Pediatr*. 2010; 157: 85–91.

Sahin F, et al. Screening for developmental dysplasia of the hip: Results of a 7-year follow-up study. *Pediatr Int*. 2004; 46: 162–66.

Dogruel H, et al. Clinical examination versus ultrasonography in detecting developmental dysplasia of the hip. *Int Orthop*. 2008; 32: 415–19.

Kremli MK, et al. The pattern of developmental dysplasia of the hip. *Saudi Med J*. 2003; 24: 1118–20.

Kutlu A, et al. Congenital dislocation of the hip and its relation to swaddling used in Turkey. *J Pediatr Orthop*. 1992; 12: 598–602.

Mahan ST, Kasser JR. Does swaddling influence developmental dysplasia of the hip? *Pediatrics.* 2008; 121: 177–78.

Swaddling: IHDI position statement. International Hip Dysplasia website. http://www.hipdysplasia.org/For-Physicians /Pediatricians/default.aspx.

Price CT, Schwend RM. Improper swaddling a risk factor for developmental dysplasia of hip. *AAP News.* September 1, 2011. http://aapnews.aappublications.org/content/32/9/11.1.full

Vennemann MM et al. sleep environment risk factors for sudden infant death syndrome: The German sudden infant death syndrome study. *Pediatrics.* 2009; 123: 1162.

L'Hoir MP, et al. Risk and preventive factors for cot death in the Netherlands, a low-incidence country. *Eur J Pediatr* 1998; 157: 681–88.

Wilson CA, Taylor BJ, Laing RM, et al. Clothing and bedding and its relevance to sudden infant death syndrome: Further results from the New Zealand cot death study. *J Paediatr Child Health.* 1994; 30: 506–12.

Ponsonby, A, et al. Factors potentiating the risk of sudden infant death syndrome associated with the prone position. *N Engl J Med.* 1993; 329: 377–82.

Blair PS, et al. Hazardous cosleeping environments and risk factors amenable to change: case-control study of SIDS in south west England. *BMJ.* 2009; 339: b3666.

McDonnell E, Moon RY. Infant deaths and injuries associated with wearable blankets, swaddle wraps, and swaddling. *J Pediatr.* 2014; 164: 1152–56.

Lipton E, et al. Swaddling, a child care practice: Historical, cultural and experimental observations. *Pediatrics.* 1965; 35 (Sup): 521–67.

Gerard CM, Harris KA, Thach BT. Physiologic studies on swaddling: An ancient childcare practice, which may promote the supine position for infant sleep. *J Pediatr.* 2002; 141: 398–404.

Gerard C, et al, Spontaneous arousals in supine infants while swaddled and unswaddled during rapid eye movement and quiet sleep. *Pediatrics.* 2002; 110: e70.

Franco P, et al. Influence of swaddling on sleep and arousal characteristics of healthy infants. *Pediatrics.* 2005; 115: 1307–11.

Narangerel G, et al. The effects of swaddling on oxygen saturation and respiratory rate of healthy infants in Mongolia. *Acta Paediatr.* 2007; 96: 261–65.

Richardson H, et al. Minimizing the risks of sudden infant death syndrome: To swaddle or not to swaddle? *J Pediatr.* 2009; 155: 475–81.

Manaseki-Holland S, et al. Effects of traditional swaddling on development: A randomized controlled trial. *Pediatrics.* 2010; 126: e1453–60.

Dennis CL, Ross L. Relationship among infant sleep patterns, maternal fatigue and development of depressive symptomatology. *Birth.* 2005; 32: 187–93.

Dørheim SK, et al. Sleep and depression in postpartum women: A population-based study. *Sleep.* 2009; 32: 847–55.

Swanson LM, et al. Relationships among depression, anxiety, and insomnia symptoms in perinatal women seeking mental health treatment. *J Womens Health.* 2011: 20; 553–58.

Paulson JF, et al. Prenatal and postpartum depression in fathers and its association with maternal depression: A meta-analysis. *JAMA.* 2010; 303: 1961–69.

Vik T, et al. Infantile colic, prolonged crying and maternal postnatal depression. *Acta Paediatr.* 2009; 98: 1344–48.

Maxted AE, et al. Infant colic and maternal depression. *Infant Ment Health J.* 2005; 26: 56–68.

Radesky J et al. Inconsolable infant crying and maternal postpartum depressive symptoms. *Pediatrics.* 2013; 131: 1–8.

Meyer LE, Erler T. Swaddling: a traditional care method rediscovered. *World J Pediatr.* 2011; 7: 155–60.

Spencer JAD, et al. White noise and sleep induction. *Arch Dis Child.* 1990; 65: 135–37.

Symon B, et al. Reducing postnatal depression, anxiety and stress using an infant sleep intervention. *BMJ Open* 2012; 2: e00166.

Harrington J, et al. Effective analgesia using physical interventions for infant immunizations. *Pediatrics.* 2012; 129: 815–22.

Personal communication—William Meyer, Ph.D., Durham, N.C.

Johannes B, Menei L. Calming techniques ease mother's minds. *Spectrum Nursing Magazine.* March 28, 2007.

St. James-Roberts I, Halil T: Infant crying patterns in the first year: Normal community and clinical findings. *J Child Psychol Psychiatry.* 1991; 32: 951–68.

Sutphen J. Is it colic or is it gastroesophageal reflux? *J Pediatr Gastroenterol Nutr.* 2001; 33: 110–11.

2004 Sleep in America Poll Final Report. National Sleep Foundation. March 2004. http://www.sleepfoundation.org /sites/default/files/2004SleepPollFinalReport.pdf

Barr RG, et al. Age-related incidence curve of hospitalized Shaken Baby Syndrome cases: Convergent evidence for crying as a trigger to shaking, *Child Abuse Negl.* 2006; 30: 7–16.

Taheri S, et al. Short sleep duration is associated with reduced leptin, elevated ghrelin, and increased body mass index (BMI). *Sleep.* 2004; 27: A146–47.

Paul IM, et al. Preventing obesity during infancy: A pilot study. *Obesity.* 2011; 19: 353–61.

Wolff, PH. The causes, controls, and organization of behavior in the neonate. *Psychol Issues.* 1966; 5: 1–105.

American Academy of Pediatrics. *Caring for Our Children: National Health and Safety Performance Standards; Guidelines for Early Care and Education Programs.* 3rd ed. Elk Grove Village, IL: American Academy of Pediatrics; 2011.

Task Force on Sudden Infant Death Syndrome. SIDS and other

sleep-related infant deaths: Expansion of recommendations
for a safe infant sleeping environment. 2011; *Pediatrics*.
128: e1341–67.

Shelov SP. *Caring for Your Baby and Young Child: Birth to Age Five*.
5th ed. New York: Bantam Books; 2009.

Karp H. "Swaddling: Boosts babies' sleep, stops colic, and reduces
infant risks." Swaddling Research. http://www.healthychildren
.org/English/tips-tools/Symptom-Checker/Pages/Crying
-Baby-Less-Than-3-Months-Old.aspx.

American Academy of Pediatrics website. http://www2.aap.org
/sections/scan/practicingsafety/toolkit_resources/module1
/swaddling.pdf

Li DK, et al. Infant sleeping position and the risk of sudden infant
death syndrome in California, 1997–2000. *Am J Epidemiol*.
2003; 157: 446–55.

Vennemann MM, et al. Sleep environment risk factors for sudden
infant death syndrome: The German sudden infant death
syndrome study. *Pediatrics*. 2009; 123: 1162–70.

Richardson HL, et al. Minimizing the risks of sudden infant
death syndrome: To swaddle or not to swaddle? *J Pediatr*. 2009;
155: 475–81.

Franco P, et al. Influence of swaddling on sleep and arousal
characteristics of healthy infants. *Pediatrics*. 2005; 115: 1307–11.

Yurdakok K, et al. Swaddling and acute respiratory infections. *Am J
Public Health*. 1990; 80: 873–75.

Manaseki-Holland S. Investigation of the Effect of Swaddling on
Lower Respiratory Tract Infection in Infants From Mongolia
[Ph.D. thesis]. London, UK: London University; 2005. http://
webcache.googleusercontent.com/search?q=cache
:pNNAhkl4-B0J: www.countdown2015mnch.org
/2005conference/alldocs/S+Manaseki-Holland.doc+swaddle
+respiratory+infection+manaseki&hl=en&gl=us.

McDonnell E, Moon RY. Infant deaths and injuries associated with wearable blankets, swaddle wraps, and swaddling. *J Pediatr.* 2014; 164: 1152–56.

Gregg CL, et al. The relative efficacy of vestibular-proprioceptive stimulation and the upright position in enhancing visual pursuit in neonates. Child Dev. 1976; 47: 309–14.

Campos RG. Rocking and pacifiers: Two comforting interventions for heelstick pain. *Res Nurs Health.* 1994; 17; 321–31.

Giacoman SL. Hunger and motor restraint on arousal and visual attention in the infant. *Child Dev.* 1971; 42: 605–14.

Chapter 9. 2nd *S*: Side/Stomach—Your Baby's Feel-Good Position

Shapiro-Mendoza CK, et al. US infant mortality trends attributable to accidental suffocation and strangulation in bed from 1984 through 2004: Are rates increasing? *Pediatrics.* 2009; 123: 533–39.

Holt LE. *The Care and Feeding of Children: A Catechism for the Use of Mothers and Nurses.* New York: D. Appleton; 1894:66.

Hunziker U, Barr R: Increased carrying reduces infant crying: A randomized controlled trial. *Pediatrics.* 1986; 77:641.

St James-Roberts I, Bowyer J, Hurry J, et al. Supplementary carrying compared with advice to increase responsive parenting as interventions to prevent persistent crying. *Pediatrics.* 1995; 95: 381–88.

Barr RG, McMullan SJ, Speiss H, et al. Carrying as colic "therapy": A randomized, controlled study. *Pediatrics.* 1991; 87: 623–30.

Baddock SA, et al. Differences in infant and parent behaviors during routine bed sharing compared with cot sleeping in the home setting. *Pediatrics.* 2006; 117: 1599–607.

Chapter 10. 3rd *S*: Shushing—Your Baby's Favorite Soothing Sound

Walker D, et al. Intrauterine noise: A component of the fetal environment. *Am J Obstet Gynecol.* 1971; 109: 91–95.

Smith CV, et al. Intrauterine sound levels: Intrapartum assessment

with an intrauterine microphone. *Am J Perinatol.* 1990;
7: 312–15.

Brackbill Y, et al. Arousal level in neonates and preschool children
under continuous auditory stimulation. *J Exp Child Psychol.*
1966; 4: 178–88.

Smith CR, Steinschneider A. Differential effects of prenatal
rhythmic stimulation on neonatal arousal states. *Child Dev.*
1975; 46: 574–78.

Birns B, Blank M, Bridger WH, et al. Behavioral inhibition in
neonates produced by auditory stimulation. *Child Dev.* 1965;
36: 639–45.

Brackbill Y. Continuous stimulation and arousal levels in infancy:
effects of stimulus intensity and stress. *Child Dev.* 1975;
46: 364–69.

Hugh, SC, et al. Infant sleep machines and hazardous sound
pressure levels. *Pediatrics.* 2014; 133: 677–81.

Karakoç A, Türker F. Effects of White Noise and Holding on Pain
Perception in Newborns. *Pain Manag Nurs.* 2014; 15: 864–70.

Sanes DH, Bao S. Tuning up the developing auditory CNS. *Curr
Opin Neurobiol.* 2009; 19: 188–99.

Chang EF, et al. Environmental noise retards auditory cortical
development. *Science.* 2003; 300: 498.

Zhang LI, et al. Disruption of primary auditory cortex by
synchronous auditory inputs during a critical period. *Proc Natl
Acad Sci USA.* 2002; 99: 2309–14.

Chapter 11. 4th *S*: Swinging—Moving in Rhythm with Your Baby

Holt LE. *The Care and Feeding of Children: A Catechism for the
Use of Mothers and Nurses.* New York: D. Appleton; 1894:66.

van den Daele L. Modification of infant state by treatment in a
rockerbox. *J Psychol.* 1970; 74: 161–65.

Brackbill Y. Continuous stimulation reduces arousal level: stability
of the effect over time. *Child Dev.* 1973; 44: 43–46.

Pederson DR, et al. The influence of amplitude and frequency of vestibular stimulation on the activity of 2-month-old infants. *Child Dev.* 1973; 44: 122–28.

Koner A, et al. The relative efficacy of contact and vestibulo-proprioceptive stimulation in soothing neonates. *Child Dev.* 1972; 43: 443–53.

Pederson DR. The soothing effect of rocking as determined by direction and frequency of movement. *Can J Behav Sci.* 1975; 7: 237–43.

Harrington J, et al. Effective analgesia using physical interventions for infant immunizations. *Pediatrics.* 2012; 129: 815–22.

Reijneveld SA, et al. Infant crying and abuse. *Lancet.* 2004; 364: 1340–42.

American Academy of Pediatrics. Shaken baby syndrome: Rotational cranial injuries—technical report. *Pediatrics.* 2001; 108: 206–10.

Catherine N, et al. Should we do more to get the word out? Causes of, responses to, and consequences of crying and colic in popular parenting magazines. *J Dev Behav Pediatr.* 2005; 26: 14–23.

Theodore A, et al. Epidemiological features of the physical and sexual maltreatment of children in the Carolinas. *Pediatrics.* 2005; 115: 331–37.

Barr RG, et al. Age-related incidence curve of hospitalized Shaken Baby Syndrome cases: Convergent evidence for crying as a trigger to shaking, *Child Abuse Negl.* 2006; 30: 7–16.

Talvik I, et al. Shaken baby syndrome and a baby's cry. *Acta Paediatr.* 2008; 97: 782–85.

American Academy of Pediatrics website. http://www2.aap.org/sections/scan/practicingsafety/toolkit_resources/module1/swadling.pdf

Child Abuse and Neglect: An Introductory Manual for Professionals and Paraprofessionals. Colorado Department of Public Health and Environment. 2006.

Pennsylvania American Academy of Pediatrics. Crying Card.
2007. http://www.pascan.org/pdf/crying_card_eng.pdf

National Association of Children's Hospitals and Related
Institutions. Profile Series. Children's Hospitals at the
Frontlines: The Prevention of Child Abuse and Neglect. 2007.

Chapter 12. 5th *S*: Sucking—The Icing on the Cake

Harrington J, et al. Effective analgesia using physical interventions
for infant immunizations. *Pediatrics.* 2012; 129: 815–22.

Campos RG. Rocking and pacifiers: Two comforting interventions
for heelstick pain. *Res Nurs Health.* 1994; 17: 321–31.

Woodson R, et al. Effects of nonnutritive sucking on state and
activity: Term-preterm comparisons. *Infant Behav Dev.* 1985;
8: 435–41.

Campos RG. Soothing pain-elicited distress in infants with
swaddling and pacifiers. *Child Dev.* 1989; 60: 781–92.

Hauck, FR, et al. Do pacifiers reduce the risk of sudden infant
death syndrome? A meta-analysis. *Pediatrics.* 2005;
116: e716–e723.

Hesselmar B, et al. Pacifier cleaning practices and risk of allergy.
Pediatrics. 2013; 131: 1–9.

Howard CR, et al. Randomized clinical trial of pacifier use and
bottle-feeding or cupfeeding and their effect on breastfeeding.
Pediatrics. 2003; 111: 511–18.

Jaafar SH, et al. Effect of restricted pacifier use in breastfeeding
term infants for increasing duration of breastfeeding. *Cochrane
Database Syst Rev.* 2012; 7.

Pickler RH, et al. The Effect of Nonnutritive Sucking on Bottle
Feeding Stress in Preterm Infants. *J Obstet Gynecol Neonatal
Nurs.* 2003; 22: 230–34.

Niemelä M, et al. A pacifier increases the risk of recurrent acute
otitis media in children in day care centers. *Pediatrics.* 1995;
96: 884–88.

Barr RG, Konner M, et al. Crying in !Kung San infants: A test of the cultural specificity hypothesis. *Dev Med Child Neurol.* 1991; 33: 601–10.

McDonnell, E, Moon, RY. Infant deaths and injuries associated with wearable blankets, swaddle wraps, and swaddling. *J Pediatr.* 2014; 164: 1152–56.

Kair LR, et al. Pacifier restriction and exclusive breastfeeding. *Pediatrics.* 2013; 131: e1101–7.

Illingsworth R. The 3-months colic. *Arch Dis Child.* 1954; 29: 165.

Kendall-Tackett K, et al. Mother-infant sleep locations and nighttime feeding behavior: U.S. Data from the survey of mothers' sleep and fatigue. *Clin Lact.* 2010; 1: 27–31.

Van Dongen HPA, et al. The cumulative cost of additional wakefulness: dose-response effects on neurobehavioral functions and sleep physiology from chronic sleep restriction and total sleep deprivation. *Sleep.* 2003; 2: 117–26.

Ball H. Airway covering during bed-sharing. *Child Care Health Dev.* 2009; 35: 728–37.

Baddock SA, et al. Differences in infant and parent behaviors during routine bed sharing compared with cot sleeping in the home setting. *Pediatrics.* 2006; 117: 1599–607.

Chapter 13. The Cuddle Cure: Finding Your Baby's Favorite Mix of S's

Brackbill, Y. Cumulative effects of continuous stimulation on arousal levels in infants. *Child Dev.* 1971; 42: 17–26.

Brackbill Y. Continuous stimulation reduces arousal level: Stability of the effect over time. *Child Dev.* 1973; 44: 43–46.

Gregg C, et al. The relative efficacy of vestibular-proprioceptive stimulation and the upright position in enhancing visual pursuit in neonates. *Child Dev.* 1976; 47: 309–14.

Gatts JD, et al. Reducing crying and irritability in neonates using a continuously controlled early environment. *J Perinatol.* 1995; 15: 215–21.

Kramer LI, Pierpont ME. Rocking waterbeds and auditory stimuli to enhance growth of preterm infants. *J Pediatr.* 1976; 88: 297–99.

Konner M. Aspects of the developmental ethnology of a foraging people. In: NG Blurton-Jones, ed. *Ethnological Studies of Child Behaviour.* New York: Cambridge University Press; 1972: 285–304.

Chapter 14. Other Colic Remedies: From Old Wives' Tales to Proven Soothers

Field T, et al. Preterm infant massage therapy research: A review. *Infant Behav Dev.* 2010; 33: 115–24.

Field, T, et al. Pregnant women benefit from massage therapy. *J Psychosom Obstet Gynaecol.* 1999; 20: 31–38.

Tiffany Field. *Touch and Massage in Early Child Development.* Johnson & Johnson Pediatric Institute; 2004.

Vandenplas Y, et al. Guidelines for the diagnosis and management of cow's milk protein allergy in infants. *Arch Dis Child.* 2007; 92: 902–8.

Hall B, et al. Infantile colic: A systematic review of medical and conventional therapies. *J Paediatr Child Health.* 2012; 48: 128–37.

Leung A, Otley A. Concerns for the use of soy-based formulas in infant nutrition. *Paediatr Child Health.* 2009; 14: 109–13.

Soy protein infant formulae and follow-on formulae: a commentary by the ESPGHAN Committee on Nutrition. *J Pediatr Gastroenterol Nutr.* 2006; 42: 352–61.

Taubman, B. Parental counseling compared with elimination of cow's milk or soy milk protein for the treatment of infant colic syndrome: A randomized trial. *Pediatrics.* 1988; 81: 756–61.

Thomas DW, et al. Infantile colic and type of milk feeding. *Am J Dis Child.* 1987; 141: 451–53.

Hill DJ, et. Effect of a low-allergen maternal diet on colic among breastfed infants: A randomized, controlled trial. *Pediatrics.* 2005; 116: e709–15.

Ize-Ludlow D et al. Neurotoxicities in infants seen with the consumption of star anise tea. *Pediatrics.* 2004; 114; e653.

Weizman, Z. et al. Efficacy of herbal tea preparation in infantile colic. *J Pediatr,* 1993; 122: 650–52.

Savino F, et al. A randomized double-blind placebo-controlled trial of a standardized extract of *Matricariae recutita, Foeniculum vulgare* and *Melissa officinalis* (ColiMil) in the treatment of breast-fed colicky infants. *Phytother Res.* 2005; 19: 335–40.

FDA warns consumers about the risk of cryptosporidium illness from baby's bliss gripe water. U.S. Food and Drug Administration website. http://www.fda.gov/newsevents /newsroom/pressannouncements/2007/ucm108990.htm.

$2.5 billion spent, no alternative cures found. Associated Press. June 10, 2009. http://www.nbcnews.com/id/31190909 /#.VDGqlb6WtG5.

Reinthal M, Andersson S, Gustafsson M, et al. Effects of minimal acupuncture in children with infantile colic—a prospective, quasi-randomised single blind controlled trial. *Acupunct Med.* 2008; 26: 171–82.

Aviner S, et al. Use of a homeopathic preparation for "infantile colic" and an apparent life-threatening event. *Pediatrics.* 2010; 125: e318–23.

Glatstein, MM. Choking caused by a homeopathic drug in a previously healthy infant. *Can Fam Physician.* 2013; 59: 848–51.

Chapter 15. The Magical 6th S: Sleep!

Karp H. *The Happiest Baby Guide to Great Sleep: Simple Solutions for Kids from Birth to 5 Years.* New York: William Morrow; 2013.

Tikotzky L, et al. VII. Infant Sleep Development from 3 to 6 Months Postpartum: Links with maternal sleep and paternal involvement. Monographs of the Society for Research in Child Development. 2015; 80: 107–124.

Kendall-Tackett K, et al. The effect of feeding method on sleep duration, maternal well-being, and postpartum depression. *Clinical Lactation* 2011; 2: 22-26.

Tikotzky L, et al. VII. Infant sleep development from 3 to 6 months postpartum: Links with maternal sleep and paternal involvement. Monographs for the Society for Research in Child Development. 2015; 80: 107–24.

Montgomery-Downs, HE, et al. Infant feeding methods and maternal sleep and daytime functioning. *Pediatrics.* 2010; 126: e1562–68.

Vladyslav V, et al. Local sleep in awake rats. *Nature.* 2011; 472: 443–47.

St James-Roberts I, et al. Video evidence that London infants can resettle themselves back to sleep after waking in the night, as well as sleep for long periods, by 3 months of age. *J Dev Behav Pediatr.* 2015; 36: 324–329.

Vennemann MM et al. Sleep environment risk factors for sudden infant death syndrome: The German sudden infant death syndrome study. *Pediatrics.* 2009; 123: 1162.

2004 Sleep in America Poll Final Report. National Sleep Foundation. March 2004. http://sleepfoundation.org/sleep -polls-data/sleep-in-america-poll/2004-children-and-sleep.

Colson ER, et al. Reports of Infant Sleep Behaviors from a National Sample of Mothers: The Study of Attitudes and Factors Affecting Infant Care (SAFE). Presentation, Pediatric Academic Societies, Vancouver, B.C. May 3, 2014. http://www .abstracts2view.com/pas/view.php?nu=PAS14L1_1690.4.

St James-Roberts I, et al. Infant crying and sleeping in London, Copenhagen and when parents adopt a "proximal" form of care. *Pediatrics.* 2006; 117: e1146–e1155.

Hysing M, et al. Trajectories and predictors of nocturnal

awakenings and sleep duration in infants. *J Dev and Behav Pediatr.* 2014; 35: 309–16.

Bell JF and Zimmerman FJ. Shortened nighttime sleep duration in early life and subsequent childhood obesity. *Arch Pediatr and Adolesc Med.* 2010; 164: 840–45.

Meyer LE, Erler T. Swaddling: A traditional care method rediscovered. *World J Pediatr.* 2011; 7: 155–60.

Manaseki-Holland S, et al. Tracking Progress in Maternal, Newborn and Child Health. Countdown to 2015; Maternal, Newborn & Child Survival. Washington, DC; June 7– 9, 2010.

Paul IM, et al. Preventing obesity during infancy: A pilot study. *Obesity.* 2011; 19: 353–61.

Franco P, et al. Influence of swaddling on sleep and arousal characteristics of healthy infants. *Pediatrics.* 2005; 115: 1307–11.

Richardson HL, et al. Minimizing the risks of sudden infant death syndrome: To swaddle or not to swaddle? *J Pediatr.* 2009; 155: 475–81.

Willinger, M. et al. Factors associated with caregivers' choice of infant sleep position, 1994–1998: The national infant sleep position study. *JAMA.* 2000; 283: 2135–42.

Colson E, et al. Trends and factors associated with infant sleeping position: The national infant sleep position study, 1993–2007. *Arch Pediatr Adolesc Med.* 2009; 163: 1122–28.

van Sleuven B, et al: Comparison of behavior modification with/ without swaddling as interventions for excessive cry. *J Pediatr.* 2006; 149: 512–17.

Gerard CM, et al. Physiologic studies on swaddling: An ancient child care practice, which may promote the supine position for infant sleep. *J Pediatr.* 2002; 141: 398–40.

Gerard CM, et al. Spontaneous arousals in supine infants while swaddled and unswaddled during rapid eye movement and quiet sleep. *Pediatrics.* 2002; 110: 6.

Oden RP, et al. Swaddling: Will it get babies onto their backs for sleep? *Clin Pediatr (Phila).* 2012; 51: 254–59.

Vennemann MM, et al. Sleep environment risk factors for sudden infant death syndrome: The German sudden infant death syndrome study. *Pediatrics.* 2009; 123: 1162–70.

Hugh, SC, et al. Infant sleep machines and hazardous sound pressure levels. *Pediatrics.* 2014; 133: 677–81.

Spencer JAD, Moran DJ, Lee A, et al. White noise and sleep induction. *Arch Dis Child.* 1990; 65: 135–37.

van der Wal, MF, et al. Mothers' reports of infant crying and soothing in a multicultural population. *Am J Dis Child.* 1998; 79: 312–17.

Willinger, M. et al. Factors associated with caregivers' choice of infant sleep position, 1994–1998. The national infant sleep position study. *JAMA.* 2000; 283: 2135–42.

Oden RP, et al. Swaddling: Will it get babies onto their backs for sleep? *Clin Pediatr.* 2012; 51: 254–59.

Pinilla T, Birch LL. Help me make it through the night: Behavioral entrainment breast-fed infants' sleep patterns. *Pediatrics.* 1993; 91: 436–44.

Shapiro-Mendoza CK, et al. US infant mortality trends attributable to accidental suffocation and strangulation in bed from 1984 through 2004: Are rates increasing? *Pediatrics.* 2009; 123: 533–39.

Colson ER, et al. Reports of Infant Sleep Behaviors from a National Sample of Mothers: The Study of Attitudes and Factors Affecting Infant Care (SAFE). Presentation, Pediatric Academic Societies, Vancouver, B.C., May 3, 2014. http://www.abstracts2view.com/pas/view.php?nu=PAS14L1_1690.4.

Colvin JD et al. Sleep environment risks for younger and older infants. *Pediatrics.* 2014; 134: e406–12.

Child Health USA 2013 website. http://mchb.hrsa.gov/chusa13/perinatal-health-status-indicators/pdf/ss.pdf.

Cote A, et al. Sudden infant deaths in sitting devices. *Arch Dis Child.* 2008; 93: 384–89.

Blair PS, et al. Hazardous cosleeping environments and risk factors amenable to change: Case-control study of SIDS in southwest England. *BMJ.* 2009; 339: b3666.

Kendall-Tackett K, et al. Mother-infant sleep locations and nighttime feeding behavior: U.S. data from the survey of mothers' sleep and fatigue. *Clin Lact.* 2010; 1: 27–31.

Willinger, M. et al. Factors Associated With Caregivers' Choice of Infant Sleep Position, 1994–1998. The National Infant Sleep Position Study. *JAMA.* 2000; 283: 2135–42.

Colson E, et al. Trends and factors associated with infant sleeping position: The national infant sleep position study, 1993–2007 *Arch Pediatr Adolesc Med.* 2009; 163: 1122–28.

Vennemann MM, et al. Sleep environment risk factors for sudden infant death syndrome: The German sudden infant death syndrome study. *Pediatrics.* 2009; 123: 1162–70.

Colson ER, et al. Reports of Infant Sleep Behaviors from a National Sample of Mothers: The Study of Attitudes and Factors Affecting Infant Care (SAFE). Presentation, Pediatric Academic Societies, Vancouver, BC. May 3, 2014. http://www .abstracts2view.com/pas/view.php?nu=PAS14L1_1690.4.

SIDS/SUID. Child Health USA 2013 website. http://mchb.hrsa .gov/chusa13/perinatal-risk-factors-behaviors/p/safe-sleep -behaviors.html.

Trends and factors associated with bed-sharing: The national infant sleep position study 1993–2010. *JAMA Pediatr.* 2013; 167: 1032–37. http://www.ncbi.nlm.nih.gov/pmc/articles /PMC3903787/figure/F1/.

St James-Roberts I, et al. Infant crying and sleeping in London, Copenhagen and when parents adopt a "proximal" form of care. *Pediatrics.* 2006; 117: e1146–55.

Hysing M, et al. Trajectories and predictors of nocturnal

awakenings and sleep duration in infants. *J Dev Behav Pediatr.* 2014; 35: 309–16.

Teti DM, et al. Marital and emotional adjustment in mothers and infant sleep arrangements during the first six months. Monographs of the Society for Research in Child Development. 2015; 80:160–176.

Baddock SA, et al. Differences in infant and parent behaviors during routine bed sharing compared with cot sleeping in the home setting. *Pediatrics.* 2006; 117: 1599–607.

Vennemann MM, et al. Sleep environment risk factors for sudden infant death syndrome: The German sudden infant death syndrome study. *Pediatrics.* 2009; 123: 1162–70.

Ruys JH, et al. Bedsharing in the first four months of life: A risk factor for sudden infant death. *Acta Paediatr.* 2007; 96: 1399–403.

Carpenter, Robert, et al. Bed sharing when parents do not smoke: Is there a risk of SIDS? An individual level analysis of five major case–control studies. *BMJ Open.* 2013; 3: e002299.

Colvin JD et al. Sleep environment risks for younger and older infants. *Pediatrics.* 2014; 134: e406–12.

Willinger, M. et al. Factors associated with caregivers' choice of infant sleep position, 1994–1998: The national infant sleep position study. *JAMA.* 2000; 283: 2135–42.

Colson E, et al. Trends and factors associated with infant sleeping position: The national infant sleep position study, 1993–2007. *Arch Pediatr Adolesc Med.* 2009; 163: 1122–28.

Von Kohorn I, et al. Influence of prior advice and beliefs of mothers on infant sleep position. *Arch Pediatr Adolesc Med.* 2010; 164: 363–69.

Task Force on Sudden Infant Death Syndrome. SIDS and other sleep-related infant deaths: Expansion of recommendations for a safe infant sleeping environment. 2011; *Pediatrics.* 128: e1341–67.

Ball HL, Volpe LE. Sudden infant death syndrome (SIDS) risk reduction and infant sleep location—moving the discussion forward. *Soc Sci Med.* 2013; 79: 84–91.

Nelson EAS, et al. International child care practices study: Infant sleeping environment. *Early Hum Dev.* 2001; 62: 43–55.

Blair PS, et al. Bed-sharing in the absence of hazardous circumstances: Is there a risk of sudden infant death syndrome? An analysis from two case-control studies conducted in the UK. *PLoS One.* 2014; 9: e107799.

Rechtman LR, et al. Sofas and infant mortality. *Pediatrics.* 2014; 134: e1293–300.

Kendall-Tackett K, et al. Mother-infant sleep locations and nighttime feeding behavior: U.S. Data from the survey of mothers' sleep and fatigue. *Clinical Lact.* 2010; 1: 27–31.

Vennemann, MM, et al. Does breastfeeding reduce the risk of sudden infant death syndrome? *Pediatrics.* 2009; 123: e406–10.

Hauck FR et al. Breastfeeding and reduced risk of sudden infant death syndrome: A meta-analysis. *Pediatrics.* 2011; 128: 103–10.

Colson ER, et al. Reports of Infant Sleep Behaviors from a National Sample of Mothers: The Study of Attitudes and Factors Affecting Infant Care (SAFE). Presentation, Pediatric Academic Societies, Vancouver, BC. May 3, 2014. http://www.abstracts2view.com/pas/view.php?nu=PAS14L1_1690.4.

SIDS/SUID. Child Health USA 2013 website. http://mchb.hrsa.gov/chusa13/perinatal-risk-factors-behaviors/p/safe-sleep-behaviors.html.

Trends and factors associated with bed-sharing: The national infant sleep position study 1993–2010. *JAMA Pediatr.* 2013; 167: 1032–37. http://www.ncbi.nlm.nih.gov/pmc/articles/PMC3903787/figure/F1/.

Dørheim SK, et al. Sleep and depression in postpartum women: a population-based study. *Sleep.* 2009; 32: 847–55.

Montgomery-Downs, HE, et al. Infant feeding methods and maternal sleep and daytime functioning. *Pediatrics*. 2010; 126: e1562–68.

Kendall-Tackett K, et al. Mother-infant sleep locations and nighttime feeding behavior: U.S. Data from the survey of mothers' sleep and fatigue. *Clin Lact*. 2010; 1: 27–31.

Vyazovskiy VV, et al. Local sleep in awake rats. *Nature*. 2011; 472: 443–47.

Van Dongen HPA, et al. The cumulative cost of additional wakefulness: Dose-response effects on neurobehavioral functions and sleep physiology from chronic sleep restriction and total sleep deprivation. *Sleep*. 2003; 26: 117–29.

2004 Sleep in America Poll Final Report. National Sleep Foundation. March 2004. http://sleepfoundation.org/sleep -polls-data/sleep-in-america-poll/2004-children-and-sleep.

Baddock SA, et al. Differences in infant and parent behaviors during routine bed sharing compared with cot sleeping in the home setting. *Pediatrics*. 2006; 117: 1599–607.

Ball H. Airway covering during bed-sharing. *Child Care Health Dev*. 2009; 35: 728–37.

Bedsharing and SIDS: The whole truth. Evolutionary Parenting website. May 29, 2011. http://evolutionaryparenting.com /bedsharing-and-sids-the-whole-truth/.

Blair PS, et al. Bed-sharing in the absence of hazardous circumstances: Is there a risk of sudden infant death syndrome? An analysis from two case-control studies conducted in the UK. *PLoS One*. 2014; 9: e107799.

Blabey, MH, Gessner BD. Infant bed-sharing practices and associated risk factors among births and infant deaths in Alaska. *Public Health Rep*. 2009; 124: 527.

Vennemann MM, et al. Sleep environment risk factors for sudden infant death syndrome: The German sudden infant death syndrome study. *Pediatrics*. 2009; 123: 1162–70.

Births: Final Data for 2007. *Natl Vital Stat Rep.* August 9, 2010. http://www.cdc.gov/nchs/data/nvsr/nvsr58/nvsr58_24.pdf.

Damato EG, Burant C. Sleep patterns and fatigue in parents of twins. *J Obstet Gynecol Neonatal Nurs.* 2008; 37: 738–49.

Ball HL. Caring for twin infants: Sleeping arrangements and their implications. *Evid Based Midwifery.* 2006; 4: 10–16.

Ball HL. Together or apart? A behavioural and physiological investigation of sleeping arrangements for twin babies. *Midwifery.* 2007; 23: 404–12.

Appendix A. Red Flags and Red Alerts: When Should You Call the Doctor?

Barr R, St. James-Roberts I, Keefe M, eds. New Evidence on Unexplained Early Infant Crying: Its Origins, Nature, and Management. Johnson and Johnson Pediatric Institute, Pediatric Round Table; 2001.

Crying. Merck Manual Home Edition. http://www.merckmanuals.com/home/childrens_health_issues/symptoms_in_infants_and_children/crying.html.

Romanello S, et al. Association between childhood migraine and history of infantile colic. *JAMA.* 2013; 309: 1607–12.

Appendix B. The New Parent's Survival Guide—Ten Key Tips

Beck CT. Predictors of postpartum depression: An update. *Nurs Res.* 2001; 50: 275–85.

Dennis CL, Ross L. Relationship among infant sleep patterns, maternal fatigue, and development of depressive symptomatology. *Birth,* 2005; 32: 187–93.

Dørheim SK, et al. Sleep and depression in postpartum women: A population-based study. *Sleep.* 2009; 32: 847–55.

Vik T, et al. Infantile colic, prolonged crying, and maternal postnatal depression. *Acta Paediatr.* 2009; 98: 1344–48.

Maxted AE, et al. Infant colic and maternal depression. *Infant Ment Health J.* 2005; 26: 56–68.

Radesky J et al. Inconsolable infant crying and maternal postpartum depressive symptoms. *Pediatrics.* 2013; 131: 1–8.

Swanson LM, et al. Relationships among depression, anxiety, and insomnia symptoms in perinatal women seeking mental health treatment. *J Womens Health (Larchmt).* 2011; 20: 553–58.

Paulson JF, Bazemore SD. Prenatal and postpartum depression in fathers and its association with maternal depression: A meta-analysis. *JAMA.* 2010; 303: 1961–69.

Dear Reader,

Over the past decade, millions of parents in dozens of nations have used the 5 S's.

I hope *The Happiest Baby* tips have been helpful to you, too.

Before you know it, that tiny newborn you're cradling in your arms will blossom into a walking, talking, lightning-fast toddler. And as she starts voicing her own opinions—*between eight and twelve months*—I hope you'll take a look at *The Happiest Toddler on the Block* book and DVD. Like *The Happiest Baby,* they offer surprisingly effective tips to boost your child's confidence, patience, cooperation, and emotional happiness. These fun techniques prevent tantrums before they happen . . . and quickly soothe the ones that do occur.

The Happiest Toddler is a rich mix of brain science plus simple steps that can help your toddler . . . in a day!

> *"Dr. Karp's excellent approach makes raising toddlers a whole lot easier."*
>
> Steven Shelov, M.D., editor in chief, AAP's Caring for
> Your Baby and Young Child

> *"A joyous adventure with pearls of wisdom on every page."*
>
> Morris Green, M.D., director, Behavioral Pediatrics,
> Indiana University, Riley Hospital for Children

> *"Parents will be delighted by this clever approach to communicating with toddlers."*
>
> Janet Serwint, M.D., director, Children's Clinic,
> Johns Hopkins Medical School

Before the first birthday, you can learn to speak *Toddler-ese*—your young child's "native language"—to stop most meltdowns in a minute or less. And simple ideas such as the *fast-food rule, gossiping,* and *playing the boob* will help you turn your tot's cries of "No!" and "Don't!" into giggles and "Yes!"

My very best wishes to you for many happy years to come.

Harvey Karp, M.D.

INDEX

Page numbers of illustrations appear in italics.

ABOUT THE AUTHOR

HARVEY KARP, M.D., F.A.A.P., is an assistant professor of pediatrics at the USC School of Medicine. He is also the creator of the national bestselling DVD and book *The Happiest Toddler on the Block* and *The Happiest Baby Guide to Great Sleep: Simple Solutions for Kids from Birth to Five Years.* Thousands of specially certified *Happiest Baby* educators teach his landmark ideas on baby calming and sleep in hospitals and clinics across North America and around the world. Dr. Karp is a nationally renowned expert in child development, children's environmental health, and breast-feeding. He lives with his wife in California. His adult daughter lives in New York.

happiestbaby.com

ABOUT THE TYPE

This book was set in Horley Old Style, a typeface issued by the English type foundry Monotype in 1925. It is an old-style face, with such distinctive features as lightly cupped serifs and an oblique horizontal bar on the lowercase "e."